Clinical Information Systems

A Framework for Reaching the Vision

Ida M. Androwich, PhD, RNC, FAAN
Carol S. Bickford, PhD, RN, BC
Patricia J. Button, EdD, RN
Kathleen M. Hunter, PhD, RN, BC
Judy Murphy, BSN, RN
Joyce Sensmeier MS, RN, BC, CPHIMS

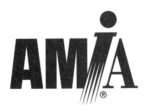

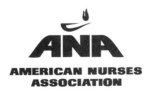

AMERICAN NURSES
ASSOCIATION

Washington, D.C.

Library of Congress Cataloging-in-Publication Data

Clinical information systems : a framework for reaching the vision
  / Ida M. Androwich ... [et al.] (American Medical Informatics
  Association, American Nurses Association).
       p. ; cm.
  Includes bibliographical references and index.
  ISBN 1-55810-206-X
  1. Nursing informatics.   I. Androwich, Ida.   II. American Medical Informatics
  Association.   III. American Nurses Association.
  [DNLM: 1. Information Systems. 2. Nursing Process. 3. Medical Informatics.
  WY 26.5 C641 2003]
  RT50.5.C556 2003
  610.73'0285—dc21

  2002152493

Published by
American Nurses Publishing
600 Maryland Avenue, SW
Suite 100 West
Washington, D.C. 20024-2571

ISBN 1-55810-206-X

CIS22   2M   12/02

Acknowledgments

In 2000, several members of the Nursing Informatics Working Group (NIWG) of the American Medical Informatics Association (AMIA) identified the need for a monograph reflecting the status of nursing information systems and providing needed follow-up to the *Next-Generation Nursing Information Systems: Essential Characteristics for Professional Practice* (Zielstorff, Hudgings, and Grobe 1993). The AMIA NIWG leadership applied for and received funding from AMIA to support the planning and writing of this new monograph. AMIA's continued support in 2001 and 2002 has ensured that the infrastructure has remained in place to support the completion of the monograph.

The authors wish to thank the following organizations for their support in the development of this monograph:

- Aurora Health Care, Milwaukee, Wisconsin
- Cerner Corporation
- Healthcare Information and Management Systems Society
- K & D Hunter Associates, Inc.
- Loyola University Chicago

Contents

Introduction | 1

Background

This monograph is the natural extension to a body of theoretical and policy work on nursing informatics begun in 1988 with the publication by the American Nurses Association (ANA) of *Computer Design Criteria for Systems That Support the Nursing Process* (Zielstorff, McHugh, and Clinton 1988). This seminal work of the ANA Council on Computer Applications in Nursing pointed out that many computer system products did not meet nursing's basic information needs. Specific criteria for designing improved systems were identified. The authors concluded with the hope that vendors and nurses would profit from the monograph's content, leading to information systems that support efficient and effective nursing care.

In 1989, the Invitational Conference on Nursing Information Systems—sponsored by the National Commission on Nursing Implementation Project (NCNIP), the ANA Council on Computer Applications in Nursing, and the National League for Nursing (NLN) Nursing Informatics Forum—brought together nursing information system (NIS) vendors and experts in nursing informatics and healthcare informatics to discuss the state of the art of information systems. The conference ended with the clear recognition that NIS vendors wanted and needed input from nurses to develop information systems and that the nursing profession had the expertise to craft recommendations that were futuristic, technologically possible, and useful to practicing nurses.

Next-Generation Nursing Information Systems: Essential Characteristics for Professional Practice (referred to hereafter as *Next-Generation*; Zielstorff, Hudgings, and Grobe 1993) is the well-known publication that synthesized the findings of the conference and other sources of contemporary thought about NISs. This monograph provided principles and guidelines that were to enable nurses and vendors to design and develop a new generation of information systems that would support the professional practice of nursing. Essential characteristics and functional requirements of this new NIS were described, along with critical information systems processes. The concept of supporting the decision-making of practicing nurses through improved information systems was strongly promoted. The authors envisioned a future in which information systems contribute to nursing's and health care's strategic goal of cost-effective, quality client care.

The authors quickly recognized that a comprehensive solution to the information management needs of clinical nurses had yet to be identified, developed, and/or implemented. The *Next-Generation* monograph provided the significant first step: identifying the solution. The authors urged that necessary resources be marshaled to develop and implement the solution. These are the second and third steps.

Today, 10 years after publication of the *Next-Generation* monograph, informatics nurses and clinical nurses still await the future(s) proposed by these important publications. The energy, enthusiasm, and knowledge of our colleagues have yet to be translated into the comprehensive NIS that supports the professional practice of nursing. However, progress is being made. Technology, nursing education, informatics research, health policy, and health economics have provided both supporting and restraining forces toward achieving the dream. As we move into the second millennium, the nursing profession in general, and informatics nurses in particular, recognize the need to revisit and rethink these original works to complete those second and third steps of the comprehensive solution advocated by Zielstorff and colleagues. This prompted members of the American Medical Informatics Association (AMIA) Nursing Informatics Working Group (NIWG) to collaborate with the ANA to craft this new monograph.

Healthcare information systems (HISs) have evolved through four phases. The first phase involved use of the financial transactions model to build the original HIS (Chu 1993). These systems supported financial, administrative, and operational transactions. In the second phase, the transactions paradigm expanded to focus on ancillary and order processing systems. The third phase incorporated data-driven systems, as described in the *Next-Generation*. This phase dramatically changed how healthcare informaticists and healthcare practitioners view data, information, and knowledge. This new monograph promotes the fourth phase, still in its beginning stages.

The fourth phase reconciles the focus on data, information, and issues related to decision-making with support of the complex, multiple flows integral to effective and efficient health care (Chu 1993; Valusek 2002). These flows focus on data, work, products, finances, clients, and so on. The fourth phase addresses these flow-driven systems within a realistic perspective. However, many vendor-developed systems still are based on the financial transactions model (Chu 1993). Some systems do address a data-driven model as described by Zielstorff and colleagues, but few have yet to deal with multiple complex flows. The data and decision-making model has achieved acceptance and at the time of its introduction was exciting. However, the reality of producing systems that support this model has been an almost insurmountable barrier (Valusek 2002).

As part of this fourth phase, healthcare practitioners recognize that useful information systems foster collaboration and cooperation by bringing together and integrating all of the information so that each practitioner may determine the information needed for their practice. Creating isolated information systems for medicine, nursing, pharmacy, and other clinical specialties is neither efficient nor effective. This monograph addresses clinical information systems (CIS) from a nursing perspective.

Purpose

The purpose of this monograph is to revisit and reformulate the principles and guidelines for clinical information systems to support professional nursing practice in light of the events, learnings, and other forces of the past 10 years. The new generation of information systems must extend beyond meeting basic information needs toward providing support for professional nursing practice to improve patient outcomes.

Organizing Framework for Clinical Information Systems

In the initial work of writing this monograph, the authors identified the need for an organizing framework to support the analysis of past events and the reformatting of the principles and guidelines for a new generation of information systems. Key concepts of this framework are:

- Professional nursing practice process understanding
- Technology
- Policy, regulation, and standards
- Information systems
- Human factors
- Technology adoption
- System utilization
- Professional nursing practice

These concepts, which are interrelated in a hierarchy of influence and feedback, illustrate the quantity and complexity of factors that require consideration in the exposition of this monograph (See Figure 1-1, next page). As in all creative endeavors, our perspectives on these concepts and their relationships changed over time. These changes are described in Chapter 5.

At the base of the hierarchy are the two concepts of professional nursing practice process understanding and technology. *Professional nursing practice process understanding* is the explicit identification of related nursing activities that, when correctly performed, satisfy the nursing practice goal. This concept provides the foundation for defining the functional requirements of an information system useful for nurses.

Technology is the application of science to work, and includes physical devices, programs, and ways of organizing work. Information technology includes hardware and software such as databases, programming languages and tools, and communication protocols. Information technology enables implementation of the functional requirements that are necessary to support applications that meet the needs of nurses and other clinicians.

Policy, regulation, and standards influence all concepts in the organizing framework and may shape their manifestation at any point in time. Healthcare policy and emerging national and international standards, combined with economic forces, impact the adoption of technology and require healthcare organizations to remain responsive to continually changing requirements for capturing, storing, and communicating data.

Information systems, representing the technical implementation of functional requirements, include application features and functions as well as the interfaces by which users interact with an application. The design and implementation of information systems may influence the degree to which users adopt and utilize the system in their work. *Human factors,* defined as the set of characteristics that underlie an individual or group's interaction with a system, can also influence the extent of a system's adoption and use. Human factors also influence information system design.

Technology adoption, in this framework, is the degree of acceptance and use of an information system within the performance of professional nursing practice. The extent of technology adoption influences the scope and depth of system utilization by individuals and organizations. *System utilization,* in turn, determines and impacts the data and information derived from the information system. *Data and information about professional nursing practice* informs and enhances our understanding of the processes of professional nursing practice. System utilization

Figure 1-1. Organizing Framework for Clinical Information Systems: Information Flow and Concept Relationships

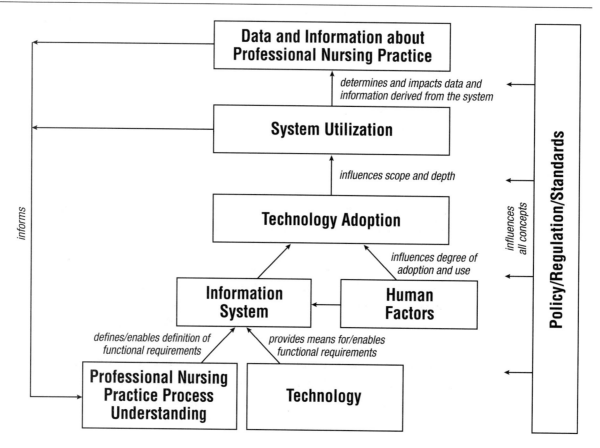

and the data and information derived from an information system also support validation of current knowledge and facilitate the synthesis of new knowledge.

Achieving the Purpose

When studying the past, this organizing framework assists in explaining the present and providing a new vision for the future in clinical information systems. This monograph also identifies reasons why the original visions of Zielstorff and her colleagues have not been achieved.

A discussion of past assumptions and expectations for clinical information systems helps to build understanding of the challenges that have impeded progress. A description follows of how the current environments for health care, information technologies, politics, economics, consumers, and other factors are influencing information system development and implementation. Using this knowledge of the past and the present, the authors identify what has impeded reaching the *Next-Generation* vision and why it has not been achieved. They explore significant elements, forces, and environmental factors, identify what has been learned about what is and is not important for CIS development and implementation, and what now needs to be done. Through analysis and reflections, the authors craft a new vision, a new framework, and a new set of recommendations.

Monograph Organization

The monograph is organized into the following sections:

1. Introduction
2. Assumptions of the Past
3. Today's Environment
4. Implications
5. Vision and Recommendations
6. Appendices

Target Audience

This monograph is written from a nursing perspective, although the influences and needs of other healthcare practitioners are incorporated in the analyses and discussions. The target audience is broad and diverse, but all are involved to some degree in the healthcare system, the healthcare industry, or healthcare information systems. Persons who might benefit from reading this monograph include all healthcare informaticists, nursing informaticists, healthcare practitioners (from all disciplines and professions), information system developers, HIS implementers, all HIS users, healthcare facility administrators (across the continuum of care), educators and leaders of future healthcare practitioners, informatics and healthcare researchers and historians, policy makers for health care and healthcare informatics, and those involved in evaluating and/or making decisions about healthcare information systems whether they are selecting a system or determining its value to an organization.

References

Chu, S. 1993. Part 1, Clinical information systems: A fourth generation. *Nursing Management* 24(18): 59–60.

Valusek, J. R. 2002. Decision support: A paradigm addition for patient safety. *Journal of Healthcare Information Management* 16(1): 34–39.

Zielstorff, R., C. Hudgings, and S. Grobe. 1993. *Next-Generation Nursing Information Systems: Essential Characteristics for Professional Practice.* Washington, DC: American Nurses Publishing.

Zielstorff, R., M. McHugh, and J. Clinton. 1988. *Computer Design Criteria for Systems That Support the Nursing Process.* Kansas City, Mo.: American Nurses Association.

Assumptions of the Past 2

The purpose of this chapter is to describe and discuss the environment in the early 1990s as it relates to clinical information systems (CISs) and their status in supporting nursing practice. This baseline understanding of the conditions at that time will help to build an understanding of the challenges that have impeded progress toward the ideal future state. The organizing framework described in the Introduction will be used to frame this discussion of the past. Key sources of information about the environment and status of systems used as references include *Next-Generation Nursing Information Systems: Essential Characteristics for Professional Nursing Practice* (Zielstorff, Hudgings, and Grobe 1993); the Institute of Medicine's report on improving the patient record (IOM 1991); HIMSS (1990, 1991, 1992, 1993, 1994, 1995, 1996, 1997, 1998, 1999, 2000); the National Center for Nursing Research (NCNR) Expert Panel on Nursing Informatics report *Nursing Informatics: Enhancing Patient Care* (NCNR 1993); the ANA publication *Computer Design Criteria* (Zielstorff, McHugh, and Clinton 1988); analysis of papers presented at the AMIA annual meetings and other major informatics conferences, from 1990 through 2000; the Pan American Health Organization document *Building Standard-Based Nursing Information Systems* (PAHO/WHO 2001); and other published literature.

Professional Nursing Practice Process Understanding

This base concept of the framework refers to the explicit identification of the set of related nursing activities that, when correctly performed, satisfy a nursing practice goal. This explicit identification of a practice process enables definition of functional requirements of the information system. In the early 1990s, there was extensive discussion in the literature and in papers presented at major conferences regarding the importance of understanding the components of the nursing process and developing systems that support data collection related to all of its phases:

- Saba and McCormick 1986
- Saba and McCormick 2001
- NIDSEC 1997
- NI 2000
- AMIA 2001
- NCNR 1993

A number of significant nursing activities from that time all focused on the identification of the data elements that are essential to nursing practice:

- 1986—Nursing Minimum Data Set conference
- 1989—Establishment of the ANA Steering Committee on Data Bases to Support Clinical Nursing Practice
- 1991—International Council of Nurses (ICN) introduction of the International Classification for Nursing Practice
- 1992—ANA recognition of nursing informatics as a nursing speciality
- 1993—Inclusion of the ANA-recognized nursing languages in the National Library of Medicine (NLM) Unified Medical Language System (UMLS)

Yet at the same time, nursing informatics education was in its infancy. Curricular content that was designed to develop the skills needed to methodically analyze and capture the key processes of nursing practice and their associated functional requirements for information systems was not available. The first nursing informatics graduate programs were developed between 1988 and 1991 with funding support from the Division of Nursing. Significantly, in the next decade, this funding was redirected to other program areas for nurse education and only recently has again been made available to nursing informatics programs.

In 1991 the National League for Nursing (NLN) adopted a general resolution to broaden the scope of nursing informatics awareness and establish goals for informatics learning in all nursing programs. Due to the somewhat general nature of the resolution, it did not result in nursing program graduates at that time understanding the importance of and developing skills in the methodologies to define process understanding. Indeed, it was not until 1992 that the ANA recognized nursing informatics as a specialty. Following that recognition, it was an additional 2 years before the *Scope of Practice for Nursing Informatics* was published by the ANA in 1994, followed by the *Standards of Practice for Nursing Informatics* in 1995.

During this time in systems development, there was a focus on data capture rather than the support of clinical processes. In 1993, the National Center for

Nursing Research (NCNR) convened a Research Priority Expert Panel on Nursing Informatics. The panel identified the following six program goals (NCNR 1993, p. 14):

- Establish nursing language, including lexicons, classification systems, and taxonomies, as well as standards for nursing data.
- Develop methods to build databases of clinical information, including data, diagnoses, objectives, interventions and outcomes, and management information, such as staffing, charge capture, turnover, and vacancy rates; and analyze relationships among them.
- Determine how nurses use data, information and knowledge to give patient care, how care is affected by differing levels of expertise and by organizational factors and working conditions, and to design information systems accordingly.
- Develop and test decision support systems and knowledge delivery systems that are appropriate for nurses' needs.
- Develop prototypes and eventually working models of nurse workstations equipped with tools to provide nurses all the information needed for patient care, research, and education at the point of use, and linked to an integrated information system.
- Develop and implement appropriate methods to evaluate nursing information systems and applications.

Interestingly, the Research Priority Expert Panel recognized that:

> To build useful clinical tools, however, it is not enough to develop the language and structure of nursing knowledge. The tools must also be attuned to the way nurses use information and knowledge to deliver patient care. Research on clinical judgment, expertise, and decision support systems is beginning to provide evidence that nursing is characterized by unique structures and processes of judgment and decision-making. These processes need further investigation to enhance the education and professional development of nurses and foster the development of appropriate, useful decision support systems for nursing. (NCNR 1993, p.12)

The majority of identified goals, however, did not focus on process understanding.

In the early 1990s, with managed care on the horizon and cost containment a high priority, there was a strong focus on redesigning nursing care away from the primary nursing care model into a team model that included greater utilization of unlicensed assistive personnel (UAP). Therefore, the focus was on redesigning and redefining cost-effective models for delivery of nursing care at the expense of understanding the core processes of planning and delivering care. This focus on productivity was evident in the emphasis on the need for systems to measure workload and acuity and to manage nursing resources cost-effectively.

In the *Next-Generation* document, some assumptions and expectations related to professional nursing practice process understanding were identified as relevant to the requirements of systems to be developed:

- Nursing practice is essentially an information-processing activity.
- Information processing is an essential element of nursing practice.
- For the foreseeable future, nursing will continue to have multiple theoretical frameworks, lexicons, data dictionaries, and models.
- Clinical nursing will continue to have a large textual component.
- To ensure high-quality practice, nurses need access to sources of data that are beyond institutional, patient-specific data.
- Education will equip nurses to be more sophisticated in using computer technology to support delivery of care and clinical decision making.

A summary of assumptions and criteria from the *Next-Generation* document is found in Appendix A.

It is also noteworthy, that in 1988 Zielstorff and colleagues stated (Zielstorff, McHugh, and Clinton 1988, p. 2):

> The major purpose of an automated nursing information system is to support nursing activities. These activities can be classified into two major categories: interdependent functions and independent functions. Interdependent functions include all activities originating from or pertaining to other departments and disciplines, such as implementation of medical orders, documentation of business information related to admission, transfer and discharge, and communication with other disciplines and departments. Independent functions include all activities involved in applying the nursing process. The nursing process is a systematic, theoretical foundation generic to all nursing practice. Essential components of the nursing process include data collection (or client assessment), diagnosis of problems amenable to nursing intervention, establishing desired outcomes, planning interventions to attain desired outcomes, and evaluating outcomes by collecting more data. This is an iterative and ongoing process that continues throughout the course of care.

Consequently, although there was recognition of the requirement for systems to support the processes of nursing, the combination of the strong focus on data definition and collection, the early nature of informatics education, and the emphasis on system utilization for cost containment and productivity enhancement delayed the methodical definition of professional nursing practice processes and the use of this definition as a fundamental source of functional requirements for clinical information systems.

In addition, as a result of the type of systems that were available and implemented at that time, the data that were collected to inform professional nursing practice were primarily related to resource management and utilization rather than the planning and decision-making processes of nursing (see Figure 2-1). Although the *Next-Generation* work supported the notion of atomic-level patient data being collected once and used many times, clinically useful data—aggregated across patients, which would allow practice patterns to be analyzed—were simply not available (Zierstorff, Hudgings, and Grobe 1993).

Figure 2-1. Examples of Uses for Atomic-Level Patient Data Collected Once, Used Many Times

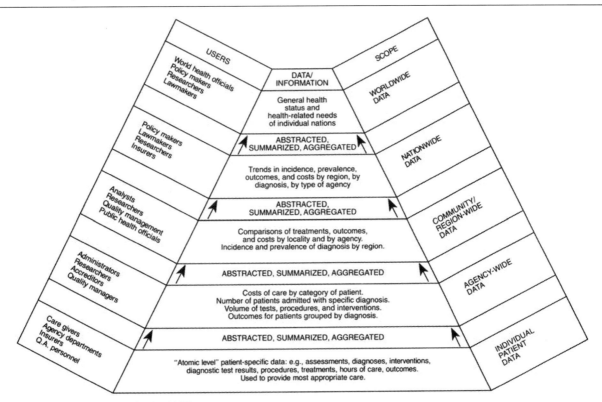

(Zielstorff, Hudgings, and Grobe 1993)

Policy, Regulation, and Standards

Policy, regulation, and standards are viewed in the organizing framework as influencing all concepts in the framework, and potentially shaping their manifestation at any point in time. Healthcare policy and emerging national and international standards, combined with economic forces, impact the adoption of technology and require healthcare organizations to remain responsive to continually changing requirements for capturing, storing, and communicating data.

In the early 1990s, the professional nursing community had already recognized the need for standards for clinical data and data communication. For example, in the *Next-Generation* (1993), two categories of standards were identified: (1) necessary vocabulary, which included data definition and (2) coding and syntax, which are concerned with the structure, communication, and transfer of data.

As mentioned, the ANA led other nursing efforts related to data standardization. In 1989, the ANA Cabinet on Nursing Practice, in response to its charge to develop policy recommendations related to the development of database systems, formed the Steering Committee on Databases to Support Clinical Nursing Practice. The mission of this committee was to accomplish the following:

- Propose policy and program initiatives regarding nursing classification schemes, uniform nursing data sets, and the inclusion of nursing data elements in national databases.
- Build national data sets for clinical nursing practice based on elements contained in standards, criteria, and guidelines.
- Coordinate ANA's initiatives related to all public and private efforts regarding the development of databases and ANA's relationship to the development and maintenance of standards, guidelines, and payment reform for nursing services.

Key contributions of the Steering Committee in the early 1990s included the committee's adoption of the Nursing Minimum Data Set (NMDS) and the committee's resultant work on recognition of nursing vocabularies, taxonomies, and classification systems for nursing practice. The criteria used in determining whether ANA would recognize a vocabulary or classification system to be used for clinical practice were developed as follows. The (terminology) system should:

- Be clinically useful for making diagnostic, intervention, and outcome decisions.
- Be stated clearly and unambiguously, with terms precisely defined.
- Have been tested for reliability of the vocabulary terms.
- Have been validated as useful for clinical purposes.
- Be accompanied by documentation of the systematic methodology used to develop the scheme.
- Be accompanied by evidence of a process for periodic review and provision for addition, revision, or deletion of terms.
- Have terms that are associated with a unique identifier or code.

It is important to note that these criteria did not address the requirements of a terminology to be incorporated in a computer-based system as defined by Cimino (1998). The absence of these criteria to drive the development of nursing languages has plagued both system developers and those trying to incorporate standardized use of nursing language in computer-based systems.

Another significant effort of ANA in supporting the definition and implementation of standards related to standardized use of nursing languages in computer-based systems was the establishment of the Nursing Information and Data Set Evaluation Center (NIDSEC[SM]) in 1996. The purpose of NIDSEC[SM] is to develop and disseminate standards pertaining to information systems that support the documentation of nursing practice and evaluate voluntarily submitted information systems against these standards. The standards used in the evaluation of information systems address five areas: standards, nomenclature, clinical content, data repository, and general systems characteristics (NIDSEC 1997).

Other key contributions related to standards during that time were the publication of the ANA *Scope of Practice for Nursing Informatics* and *Standards of*

Practice for Nursing Informatics (ANA 1994, 1995). The articulation of these standards represented progress in competency and role definition for nurses pursuing a career in nursing informatics. However, it is significant that these standards were not available until the mid-1990s. Certification in nursing informatics, offered by American Nurses Credentialing Center (ANCC), became available in the mid 1990s.

The Institute of Medicine (IOM 1991) discussed various environmental and political factors that were to influence policy and regulation. For example, an IOM committee believed that the time was ripe for strategic planning and identified five key environmental conditions that existed in the early 1990s that were likely to promote electronic patient records. These included: an increased demand for patient information throughout the healthcare sector; the development of more powerful and less expensive technologies necessary to enhance the patient record; societal (patients and providers) increase in familiarity with computers; the realities of an aging and increasingly mobile population leading to demands for portable information; and a recognition of needed reform in health care (IOM 1991).

The IOM expected that there would be barriers to the development and implementation of these systems. Barriers to development identified in 1991 included a lack of a clear definition of what a computer-based patient record (CPR) could and should be, a lack of standards for content and format of a CPR, and the inevitability of substantial costs and risks before a return on investment would be realized. Barriers to diffusion and implementation were: the U.S. healthcare system with its numerous autonomous units, its multiple reimbursement policies, and its disaggregation of care; no single organization or agency providing leadership; individual user behavior; lack of information, understanding, and awareness of the CPR; high costs of acquiring and using a CPR with few analyses existing to indicate effectiveness or benefits; formidable legal and societal issues, such as licensure, the unclear legal status of the CPR, ownership, liability for defects in systems, authentication, and privacy issues; and lack of an adequate infrastructure including network and data communication standards.

The IOM committee made a number of recommendations that they expected would effectively address the barriers to CPR implementation and use. These included: defining the CPR and its attributes as the standard for future patient records; proposing an organizational framework for systematically removing the identified barriers; identifying needed research, development, and demonstration projects; promulgation of standards for data and security; review of legal constraints; distributions of costs; and education of health professionals. The IOM committee recognized that the "challenge of coordinating the CPR development efforts in a pluralistic healthcare environment was great" (IOM 1991, p. 152), but they were convinced nevertheless that the goal of widespread use of the CPR was achievable within a decade.

Another source of data regarding expectations at that time was the Annual HIMSS Leadership Surveys that were initiated in 1990. The purpose of these surveys was to "address the technical and management issues facing members during a time of rapid technological advances in U.S. health care" (HIMSS 1990). HIMSS members include healthcare professionals in hospitals, corporate healthcare systems, clinical practice groups, healthcare information technology supplier organizations, healthcare consulting firms, and government settings in professional levels ranging from senior staff to CIOs and CEOs (see Appendix B). In these surveys, there was discussion of the anticipated impact of environmental factors and healthcare policy on information systems. In the early 1990s, survey respondents identified the need to optimize efficiency of the enterprise and contain healthcare costs as the most significant force driving computerization. And in 1993, when managed care began its influence on healthcare, respondents identified managed care as the most likely healthcare force to impact hospital investments in computer systems. Nearly two-thirds of respondents said that government and payer pressure to control costs was the greatest single force driving computerization in healthcare. In 1994 and 1995, respondents again identified the movement to managed care as the most significant force driving computerization (HIMSS 1994, 1995; see also Appendix B).

The early 1990s saw increased efforts in the definition of standards related to clinical information systems; for example, vocabulary, data communication, authentication of healthcare records, and various technologies. The focus on clinical systems integration, which was viewed as a priority in the early 1990s, drove the work of Health Level 7 in developing standards for messaging and interfacing data.

Although it was recognized that standards were important and provided potential value, in the early 1990s there were few regulations mandating the implementation of specific standards. For example, in the managed care environment, increased competition for covered lives required organizations to differentiate on basis of quality. This drove the development of systems to report quality, such as HEDIS® (Health Employer Data and Information Set), developed by the National Committee for Quality Assurance (NCQA). Also, the Joint Commission on Accreditation of Healthcare Organizations (JCAHO) in this timeframe introduced increasingly detailed requirements related to the use of information systems in healthcare organizations. This significantly impacted the acquisition and use of systems. However, for the most part, these requirements were not mandated by law.

Organizations developed local policies regarding standardized data collection without the imperative from law or government. Some state and federal mandatory reporting requirements, such as reporting of discharge information and certain claims reporting requirements, drove the development of electronic data interchange (EDI) solutions. In fact, some regulations and laws actually mitigated against automation; for example, many states lacked legal recognition of the electronic signature.

Technology

The concept of *technology* is defined in the organizing framework as the application of science to work, and includes physical devices, programs, and ways of organizing work. Information technology includes hardware and software such as databases, programming languages/tools, and communication protocols. Information technology provides the means for implementing the functional requirements necessary to support applications that meet the needs of nurses and other clinicians.

In the early 1990s, there was a consistent identification of the technologies required to develop and implement a comprehensive CPR. In addition, there was a consistent assumption that these technologies would be developed. For example, in the *Next-Generation* (Zielstorff, Hudgings, and Grobe 1993, pp. 9, 10), an explicit assumption was that "Technology will continue to evolve in ways that make information systems for professionals more useful" and that "Technologies will be developed to bridge multiple lexicons."

In the IOM report (1991), the following expectations about the technology required for implementation of the ideal patient record included:

■ Databases and database management systems
■ Workstations
■ Data acquisition and data retrieval
■ Text processing
■ Image processing and storage
■ Data exchange and vocabulary standards
■ System communications and network infrastructure
■ System reliability and security
■ Linkages to secondary databases

Results from the HIMSS surveys conducted in the early 1990s documented anticipation of the following technologies:

■ Memory storage capabilities
■ Processing power and speed
■ User interface technologies such as voice recognition, graphical user interfaces, and handwriting recognition, advances expected to increase use of systems
■ Multimedia presentations of information
■ Image processing and display
■ Miniaturization of computers and terminals
■ Connectivity among disparate systems
■ Decision support and artificial intelligence technologies

In addition, the HIMSS surveys identified the perceived importance and actual utilization of various technologies (see Table 2-1).

Throughout the early and mid 1990s, only a small percent of the nursing presentations at AMIA and other informatics conferences focused on technology or technology-related issues. (Also refer to Appendix C for a summary of 25 years of nursing informatics history; AMIA 2001.) In 1993, the NCNR Expert Panel on Nursing Informatics identified five evolving technologies that were expected to advance nursing information science and advance patient care: (1) decision support technologies (knowledge-based, model-based, and discovery methods), (2) network technologies, (3) imaging technologies, (4) real-time and time-dependent technologies, and (5) tool kit technologies (NCNR 1993).

Table 2-1. HIMSS Surveys: Perceived Importance and Actual Utilization of Various Technologies

1990–1993	Integration of existing systems was identified as the most important priority for the next 1 to 2 years.
1993	Clinical decision support was cited as the technology with the most potential for improving the quality of care in hospitals. Forty percent of respondents were moving applications off mainframes to minicomputers or personal computers and more than two-thirds were using Electronic Data Interchange (EDI) for claims processing. Open systems architecture was newly identified as a fundamental strategy.
1994	The majority of respondents considered the Internet as absolutely essential for healthcare, although fewer than half said they used it.
1994–1995	Integrating systems across facilities was identified as the most important IT priority for the next 1 to 2 years.
1995	More than one-third of institutions were using multimedia technology, primarily for education and training. Access to online healthcare information and services from home was thought to be the most significant healthcare-related computer development that would affect consumers.
1996	Smart cards were listed as the top futuristic healthcare technology expected to be in common use within 5 years. Forty-one percent of organizations used telemedicine, primarily for transmitting images of patient records. More than one-third of the organizations had developed a home page on the World Wide Web.
1997	Access to medical records via the Internet was the top futuristic healthcare technology expected to be in common use in the next 5 years

(HIMSS 1990–1997)

Finally, object-oriented modeling methodology was not widely available for use in defining the key business processes to be supported by clinical software systems in the early 1990s. Systems developed without the use of this methodology were based on assumptions of what should be done to increase efficiency, productivity, and the quality of care provided. Because no formal process existed to link systems to the processes they were intended to support, systems often missed the mark in terms of truly supporting clinical care delivery.

Information Systems

Within the framework, the concept of *information systems* is defined as encompassing application features and functions as well as the interfaces by which users interact with an application. Similar to the previously discussed status of the technology described, application features and functions and the user interface were primarily in a definitional mode as opposed to actually being executed in existing systems.

In 1988, Zielstorff, McHugh, and Clinton presented an initial identification of design criteria for automated systems to support the nursing process (see Table 2-2).

Table 2-2. Information Systems Supporting the Nursing Process: Initial Design Criteria (1988)

System capabilities

- Accommodate data elements associated with the nursing process
- Integrate with other parts of the patient record
- Eliminate need for redundant data entry
- Applications housed in system designed to facilitate info retrieval and manipulation
- Each data item defined as a key for retrieval

User-machine interface

- Flexible system to permit user tailoring to reflect conceptual framework and vocabulary in use at that site
- Permit customization of data entry formats and screens, as well as output formats
- Data entry used primarily as structured data entry formats, but with limited free text entries
- Ability to query databases without help of programmers or system analysts

Hardware requirements

- Sufficient processing power to handle calculated workload
- Response time of no greater than 2 seconds at peak usage
- Sufficient online and off-line memory for long- and short-term storage
- Enough data entry ports conveniently placed to permit rapid accessibility to all users

Data security and integrity

- Software and hardware facilities to protect security of data
- Two levels of password security
- Preserve safety and integrity of the legal record of nursing care
- Restrict power to purge record to database administration
- Permit care plans to be updated as necessary without destroying outdated information
- Back-up plans and equipment

(Zielstorff, McHugh, and Clinton 1988, pp. 10–11)

These design criteria were expanded by Zielstorff, Hudgings, and Grobe in the 1993 *Next-Generation* monograph, which identified the following assumptions and expectations regarding system features and functions (see Table 2-3).

Table 2-3. Information Systems Supporting the Nursing Process: Expanded Design Criteria (1993)

Efficiency and productivity
The system must promote efficiency and productivity.

Effectiveness of care
The system must promote effectiveness of care by assisting clinicians to make the best possible decisions for their clients.

Flexibility
- The system must be able to be configured at the implementation site with respect to conceptual framework or nursing model, structured vocabulary, displays and reports, and decision rules (p. 14).
- The system must be able to be upgraded as new technological developments become available. To every extent possible, upgrades to the system should enable transferability of existing data to the new system (p. 14).
- The system must be able to respond to changing requirements in methods of delivering care, and in methods of reporting to external agencies (p. 14).

Connectivity
- The system should be able to communicate with other information systems within the agency to reduce redundant data entry and avoid duplicate databases (p. 14).
- The system should be able to support standard and evolving communication protocols to enable data sharing among otherwise disparate systems (p. 14).
- The system should be able to provide communication links to external systems such as bibliographic retrieval systems, data banks, and other knowledge resources (p. 14).
- The system should be able to acquire data from other systems, and be able to contribute data to other systems and agencies (to support a longitudinal patient record, for example, or to contribute data to a national database for inquiry or research) (p. 14).

Performance
- The system should demonstrate satisfactory performance (according to benchmark criteria) at peak calculated workload times (p. 14).
- The system should provide continuous service (no down time), as when the system is implemented with "non-stop technology" or with redundant back-up systems (p. 14).

Security and confidentiality
- Integrity of all data should be assured, so that data are captured, transmitted, stored, and displayed without error. Mechanisms for assuring data integrity would be described and demonstrable.
- Data should be protected from unauthorized access by means of security codes and/or other unique user identifiers.
- Confidentiality of patient and provider data should be protected. There are many ways to do this. Some are as simple as not leaving a patient's data displayed on the screen for more than a certain number of seconds, unless there is verification that someone is still using it. Other methods involve more complex algorithms that either strip or encrypt unique patient and provider identifiers before sending the patient's record to a larger database for research or inquiry (p. 15).
- Audit trails should be kept of all transactions that alter data within the patient's record, including date, time, and identity of person carrying out the action. Entries subsequently marked as erroneous should be kept—not deleted—and flagged as erroneous, with the usual audit notations (p. 14).

(Page numbers refer to Zielstorff, Hudgings, and Grobe 1993)

Table 2-4. IOM Attributes of the "Ideal" Patient Record

General Attributes

Content	■ Uniform core data elements ■ Standardized coding systems and formats ■ Common data dictionary ■ Information on outcomes of care and functional status
Format	■ "Front-page" problem list ■ Ability to flip through the record ■ Integrated among disciplines
System performance	■ Rapid retrieval ■ 24-hour access ■ Available at convenient places ■ Easy data input
Linkages	■ Linkages with other information systems ■ Transferability of information among specialties and sites ■ Linkages with relevant scientific literature, other institutional databases, and registries ■ Records of family members ■ Electronic transfer of information
Intelligence	■ Decision support ■ Clinical reminders and alerts ■ "Alarm" systems capable of being customized
Reporting capabilities	■ Derived documents (insurance forms, easily customized output and user interfaces) ■ Standard clinical reports (discharge summary) ■ Customized and ad hoc reports (specific evaluation queries) ■ Trend reports ■ Graphics
Control and access	■ Easy access for patients and their advocates ■ Safeguards against violation of privacy
Training and implementation	■ Minimal training required for system use ■ Graduated implementation possible

Storage Attributes

Access	For users at any time or place in the user-preferred level of data and detail display and at a reasonable speed Recommendations for patient access were not provided
Data quality	Legibility, completeness, meaning, and accuracy; this implies systems designed to reduce errors, such as data entry screens and logical rules that: ■ flag or block inappropriate entries, ■ decrease the need for redundant data entry, and ■ accommodate the full range and complexity of clinical data.

Continued

Table 2-4. IOM Attributes of the "Ideal" Patient Record *(continued)*

Security	■ Data integrity ■ Data confidentiality
Flexibility	Customization of: ■ data entry, ■ reporting, and ■ display formats.
Connectivity	The need for any links that may improve care for the patient, such as: ■ other information databases, ■ family records, ■ links to other individuals with similar conditions/treatments for epidemiological purposes, and longitudinal record linkages.
Efficiency	■ One-time data entry ■ Automated performance of routine tasks

(IOM 1991, pp. 34, 37-46)

The IOM (1991), in its vision for clinical information systems and the computer-based patient record, identified 14 attributes of the ideal future record. It was perceived that this ideal record would be useful in meeting many stakeholder needs, such as patient care delivery, patient care support, education, research, regulation, policy, industry, and billing and reimbursement (see Table 2-4).

In addition to the storage functionality described above, it was also perceived that the ideal CPR would provide guidance for clinical problem solving, such as Weed's problem-oriented medical record (Weed 1971) and support the practitioner's knowledge base (for example, Problem-Knowledge Couplers™; Problem-Knowledge Corporation. 2002.)

Data from HIMSS surveys in the early 1990s identified that the target for greatest investment and the most important IT projects were in the area of patient care/bedside systems. There was also a focus on user interface as a priority for improvement of systems. Order entry/communications and outpatient services were the top areas for planned upgrades or implementations. By 1995, planned investments in information systems were expected to increase by 50%.

Human Factors

The concept of *human factors* is defined as the set of characteristics that underlie an individual or a group's interaction with a system. Human factors can also influence the extent of a system's design, use, and adoption.

These human factors fall into two broad categories: (1) those factors dealing with the human–computer interaction (such as interface design, terminal place, data capture methods etc.); and (2) those factors related to the change process involved in implementing computer-based systems.

In the *Next-Generation* (Zielstorff, Hudgings, and Grobe 1993, p. 15), assumptions and expectations regarding human factors fall in the first category (interface design, terminal placement, and data capture methods) and are listed as follows:

- The system must be able to accommodate a variety of data capture methods, each best suited to the circumstance and the type of data being captured. In general, the principle that data should be captured as close to the time and source of creation as possible should be followed. For some types of data, bar code readers will be most efficient; for others, touch screens, light pens, pen pads, mouse, or voice recognition will be more appropriate. Miniature hand-held terminals will be most appropriate for some tasks and settings, while laptop portable terminals may be best for others, such as home visits.

- Data capture methods must be no more time consuming than manual methods for entering comparable data. To the extent possible, the automated system should be less time consuming to use than the comparable manual system.

- The theoretical framework for the nursing process and the vocabulary to be used should be configurable at the site. Preferably, these will be determined by local professional consensus. The site should not be forced to use a particular framework simply because the system purchased is designed to work only with that framework.

- The system's user interface design should follow established principles of user–machine dialogue. Consumers may have difficulty evaluating this system characteristic. Generally, some important principles have been incorporated if the dialogue sequence seems to make sense intuitively, without a lot of explanation of what to do next; if relevant information is displayed with enough detail to inform without overwhelming at first glance; and if help and error messages are presented in clear, helpful, nonjargon phrases.

- Connections to other systems—whether internal or external to the agency— should appear seamless to the user. Incorporating all the access codes and log-on scripts within a master menu on the main system is desirable. The user would then simply choose an application and be logged on to the appropriate system.

Also in 1993, the NCNR Expert Panel in its description of the state of the science related to human factors, discussed the nursing computer workstation including physiologic aspects of the workstation and ergonomic shortcomings (strained postures, poor photometric display characteristics, inadequate lighting). The panel also noted that psychological aspects of human factors, defined as ease of use enhanced by consistent syntax and format standards across applications, had not been adequately researched. Finally, this panel identified the need for further research in workstation design incorporating ergonomic and interface design. Significantly, their recommendations did not identify the need for research about factors related to the change process involved in implementing computer-based systems (NCNR Priority Expert Panel on Nursing Informatics 1993).

The IOM (1991) defined "individual user behavior" as a barrier to CPR diffusion and implementation, but made no recommendations to address this factor (IOM 1991).

During the mid 1990s, a significant amount of time and energy began to be invested in the examination and understanding of the second category related to human factors. Those factors related to the change process involved in implementing computer-based systems.

For example, in March 1993, the International Medical Informatics Association (IMIA) sponsored a Working Group Conference on the Organizational Impact of Informatics; in September 1993, IMIA created a new working group, Organizational Impact of Medical Informatics. In 1994, the first book focused directly on these issues was published (Lorenzi and Riley 1995). And finally, in 1996, AMIA created the Organizational Aspects of Medical Informatics Working Group.

Prior to this time, although there was significant information available in the literature of a variety of disciplines about organizational change and reports of a variety of successes and failures of CIS projects, there was no organized, focused effort to address the overwhelming organizational and personal complexity of the large-scale change involved in many information system projects in health care. In 1997, Braude stated:

> The brief history of medical informatics is littered with horror stories of systems that were not completed, that were orders of magnitude over budget, or that were not used by the primary population for which they were designed. But despite the all too frequent reoccurrence of these failures, there has been little interest in looking for the reasons for them or in research into organizational impacts of change (Braude 1997, p. 150).

Technology Adoption and System Utilization

Technology adoption is defined as the degree of acceptance and use of an information system during the performance of professional nursing practice. The extent of technology adoption influences the scope and depth of system utilization by individuals and organizations. In the *Next-Generation* monograph (Zielstorff, Hudgings, and Grobe 1993), several usability principles believed to be associated with increased adoption and use of systems were identified:

- *Simple and natural dialogue.* Dialogues should not contain information that is irrelevant or rarely needed. Every extra unit of information in a dialogue competes with the relevant units of information and diminishes their relative visibility. All information should appear in a natural and logical order.
- *Speak the users' language.* The dialogue should be expressed clearly in words, phrases, and concepts familiar to the user, rather than in system-oriented terms.
- *Minimize the users' memory load.* The user should not have to remember information from one part of the dialogue to another. Instructions for use of the system should be visible or easily retrievable whenever appropriate.
- *Consistency.* Users should not have to wonder whether words, situations, and actions mean the same thing.

- *Provide feedback.* The system should always keeps users informed about what is going on through appropriate feedback within reasonable time.
- *Provide clearly marked exits.* Users often choose system functions by mistake and will need a clearly marked "emergency exit" to leave the unwanted state without having to go through an extended dialogue.
- *Provide shortcuts.* Clever shortcuts—unseen by the novice user—may often speed up the interaction for the expert user such that the system caters to both inexperienced and experienced users.
- *Good error messages.* Error messages should be expressed in plain language (no codes), precisely indicate the problem, and constructively suggest a solution.
- *Prevent errors.* Even better than good error messages is a careful design that prevents a problem from occurring in the first place.

Although there was a strong emphasis on the need for research to understand nurses' decision-making and inferences and the processes used to acquire knowledge and make clinical judgments, the NCNR document, *Nursing Informatics: Enhancing Patient Care* (1993), did not address these issues (NCNR 1993).

In the HIMSS leadership surveys, a more user-friendly user interface, voice recognition, expert systems, and handwriting recognition were named as advances in technology that were expected to increase use and adoption of systems (HIMSS 1991). In these surveys, the following was also reported about expectations and actual use of systems:

- Whereas the vast majority felt that hospitals were behind other businesses in implementing automation, one-third reported using existing computer systems to analyze clinical data to measure patient outcomes (HIMSS 1991).
- The CPR was identified as a promising concept but was thought to be 5 to 10 years away (HIMSS 1992).
- Two-thirds of respondents blended operating systems in an open systems environment and one-half were networked to physician offices for outpatient services (HIMSS 1994).

Data and Information About Professional Nursing Practice

In the late 1980s and early 1990s, there were a number of ANA initiatives related to supporting the identification and generation of data about professional nursing practice. For example, the formal recognition of Werley and Lang's Nursing Minimum Data Set (Werley and Lang 1988) took place in 1990. Throughout the 1990s there was also important definitional work actively in progress to recognize nursing vocabularies to be included in systems and to identify methods for representing nursing practice in systems not yet developed. These initiatives were previously discussed in the section related to Policy, Regulation, and Standards.

As described, there was much emphasis on system requirements to generate data and information about nursing practice. The issues that mitigated against the actual generation of such data are not unique to the United States. In 2001, PAHO, a unit of the World Health Organization (WHO), published the collective work of an international team of nursing informaticists. Included in their global level assessment of the constraints of clinical and administrative nursing documentation over the past decade were the following observations:

- The complex nature of documentation and the expansion of documentation requirements has led to increases in volume and levels of detail without a concomitant increase in the quality of the informational content.
- Data collected at other than the point-of-care requires more resources to collect, record, retrieve, and analyze and is often incomplete or missing essential detail.
- Significant and important clinical and administrative data and information are not included in individual health records.
- Intervention data are often missing, thus rendering it impossible to link nursing actions or to clarify and quantify the contribution of nursing to the health of individuals and populations.
- Specific requirements for documentation of care tend to be according to each agency, institution, level of professional education, tradition, local routine, and legal environment rather than based on standards for documentation.
- There is a lack of recognition and valuing of nursing documentation as an important aspect to explain care variation, and nursing documentation is frequently not included as a component of automated health information systems.

Thus, they conclude that documentation of nursing practice, especially nursing interventions, is one of the weakest components of the nursing care process. They identify underlying causes for this problem are "related to the insufficient numbers of providers relative to patient demands, a lack of time to record the details of the care provided and the absence of structured forms for data collection and a comprehensive system for data processing and retrieval" (PAHO/WHO 2001, p. 12).

The lack of recognition and inability to value nursing contributions related to the automated health record has been pervasive in the past. Lack of inclusion of nursing documentation in the clinical record was not even identified as an issue in the 1991 IOM report or in the HIMSS surveys. The absence of a call for documentation of nursing care cannot be blamed solely on the non-nursing world. Vendors will strive to provide that which clients demand, and nursing has not had a loud, clear, organized, or united voice to date.

Summary and Conclusion

Reflection on the discussion regarding the environment and the status of CISs in the early 1990s suggests several key themes about this time period as baseline for the monograph. First, the preponderance of available data focuses on identified expectations and requirements of what clinical systems *should* do versus data about what information systems were doing. Second, there was insufficient recognition of the fundamental need to design systems based on a solid understanding of the underlying processes to be supported. There was also a lack of methodologies necessary to enable representation and understanding of these processes as a prerequisite for system design.

Third, although there appeared to be recognition of the importance of addressing the user interface component of human factors, there was a lack of awareness not only of the available knowledge related to change management strategies for large projects, but also an apparent lack of appreciation of the fundamental importance of incorporating this knowledge into overall information system implementation strategies.

Fourth, efforts in standards development were actively underway in the early 1990s. The criteria that must underlie terminologies that are incorporated within computer-based systems were beginning to be defined. However, within nursing, the preponderance of activity was focused on definition of vocabularies and classifications that represented a significant contribution to defining terms to describe nursing, but did not meet the criteria for incorporation in computer-based systems.

Finally, in retrospect, there appears to have been an overall, naïve expectation that within the decade the healthcare industry would not only develop but also broadly implement and reap the benefit of a comprehensive, fully automated clinical record. A lack of appreciation of the significant complexity involved in both designing and implementing systems that would meet the defined expectations is apparent.

References

AMIA (American Medical Informatics Association). 2001. Panel Presentation 2001. Twenty years of nursing at SCAMC/AMIA. Paper read at AMIA Annual Meeting, November, at Washington, DC.

ANA (American Nurses Association). 1994. *The Scope of Practice of Nursing Informatics*. Washington, DC: American Nurses Publishing.

————. 1995. *Standards of Practice for Nursing Informatics*. Washington, DC: American Nurses Publishing.

Braude, R. M. 1997. People and organizational issues in health informatics. *Journal of American Medical Informatics Association* 4(2): 150–151.

Cimino, J. J. 1998. A desiderata for controlled medical vocabularies in the twenty-first century. *Methods of Information in Medicine* 37(4–5): 394–403.

HIMSS (Healthcare Information and Management Systems Society). 1990. *Annual HIMSS/Hewlett Packard Leadership Survey*. Chicago: Healthcare Information and Management Systems Society.

————. 1991. *Annual HIMSS/Hewlett Packard Leadership Survey*. Chicago: Healthcare Information and Management Systems Society.

————. 1992. *Annual HIMSS/Hewlett Packard Leadership Survey*. Chicago: Healthcare Information and Management System Society.

————. 1993. *Fourth Annual HIMSS Leadership Survey*. Chicago: Healthcare Information and Management Systems Society.

————. 1994. *Fifth Annual HIMSS Leadership Survey*. Chicago: Healthcare Information and Management Systems Society.

————. 1995. *Sixth Annual HIMSS Leadership/Hewlett Packard Survey*. Chicago: Healthcare Information and Management Systems Society.

————. 1996. *Seventh Annual HIMSS/Hewlett Packard Leadership Survey*. Chicago: Healthcare Information and Management Systems Society.

————. 1997. *Eighth Annual HIMSS/Hewlett Packard Leadership Survey*. Chicago: Healthcare Information and Management Systems Society.

————. 1998. *Ninth Annual HIMSS/Hewlett Packard Leadership Survey*. Chicago: Healthcare Information and Management Systems Society.

————. 1999. *10th Annual HIMSS/Hewlett Packard Leadership Survey*. Chicago: Healthcare Information and Management Systems Society.

————. 2000. *11th Annual HIMSS/Hewlett Packard Leadership Survey*. Chicago: Healthcare Information and Management Systems Society.

IOM (Institute of Medicine) 1991. *The Computer-based Patient Record: An Essential Technology for Change*. (R. Dick and E. Steen, authors). Washington, DC: Institute of Medicine.

International Council of Nursing. 1966. *The Classification of Nursing Practice: A Unifying Framework: The Alpha Version*. Geneva, Switzerland: International Council of Nurses.

Lorenzi, N. M., and R. T. Riley. 1995. *Organizational Aspects of Health Informatics: Managing Technological Change*. In series, *Computers in Health Care,* edited by K. Hannah, and M. Ball. New York: Springer-Verlag.

NCNR (National Center for Nursing Research). 1993. Priority Expert Panel on Nursing Informatics. *Nursing Informatics: Enhancing Patient Care*. Bethesda, MD: US Department of Health and Human Services, US Public Health Service, National Institutes of Health.

NIDSEC (Nursing Information and Data Set Evaluation Center). 1997. *Standards and scoring guidelines*. Washington, DC: American Nurses Publishing.

PAHO/WHO (Pan American Health Organization and World Health Organization.) 2001. *Building Standard-based Nursing Information Systems*. Washington, DC: PAHO Division of Health Systems Program.

Problem-Knowledge Corporation.2002. Problem-Knowledge Couplers™: Knowledge in Tools. [Cited December 2002.] URL: http://www.pkc.com.

Saba, V., and K. McCormick. 1986. *Essentials of Computers for Nursing,* 2nd ed. New York: McGraw-Hill.

———, eds. 2001. *Essentials of Computers for Nurses: Informatics for the New Millennium,* 3rd ed. New York: McGraw-Hill.

Weed, L. W. 1971. *Medical Records, Medical Education, and Patient Care*. Cleveland: The Press of Case Western Reserve University.

Werley, H., and N. Lang. 1988. The consenually derived nursing minimum data set: Elements and definitions. In *Identification of the Nursing Minimum Data Set*, edited by H. Werley, and N. Lang. New York: Springer.

Zielstorff, R., C. Hudgings, and S. Grobe. 1993. *Next-Generation Nursing Information Systems: Essential Characteristics for Professional Practice*. Washington, DC: American Nurses Publishing.

Zielstorff, R., M. McHugh, and J. Clinton. 1988. *Computer Design Criteria for Systems that Support the Nursing Process*. Kansas City, MO.: American Nurses Association.

Today's Environment 3

This chapter describes how today's environment of health care, information technology, economics, consumers, and many other factors are influencing information system development and implementation. Many of the characteristics we thought important for information systems 10 years ago no longer seem relevant today, and have been replaced by other criteria. This signals the end of the third phase (data-driven systems) and the beginning of the fourth phase (flow-driven systems) as described in the introduction to this monograph. When seeking insight and understanding of the reasons for both unmet and changing expectations for clinical information systems, it is helpful to review some key transitions that have taken place over the past decade, using the seven categories of the organizing framework:

- Professional nursing practice process understanding
- Policy, regulation, and standards
- Technology
- Information systems
- Human factors
- Technology adoption
- System utilization

An examination of the past in Chapter 2 and the current environment in this chapter set the stage for the important visioning work necessary to make recommendations for future design, development, implementation, and evaluation of clinical information systems that support nursing practice. Here, then, is a review of the seven categories and how changes in each have been influencing forces for clinical information systems' migration toward the fourth phase of flow-driven systems.

Professional Nursing Practice Process Understanding

The development of healthcare information systems in the 1990s focused initially on order communication, results reporting, ancillary department operations, diagnostic coding, and patient accounting—primarily in acute care hospital facilities. Some organizations implemented clinical documentation and care planning systems, but penetration was poor and return on investment (ROI) unclear. These systems did little to support complex care delivery activities across the continuum of care; they were often freestanding and not integrated with other healthcare information system (HIS) applications. Frequently they did not support decision-making, nor were they integrated within the workflow associated with patient care delivery processes (Ozbolt, Abraham, and Schultz, 1990). Furthermore, they did not support the prevention-wellness models characteristic of professional nursing practice outside of the acute care setting, as evidenced by infrequent and sporadic implementation in non-acute care/ambulatory settings (Staggers, Thompson, and Snyder-Halpern, 2001).

Nurses have always collected data, transforming those elements into information that then evolves into knowledge. This includes strong traditions reflected in undocumented oral stories (change-of-shift report, telephone call for patient transfer), handwritten narrative documentation, and accountability for the communication of collected information to other healthcare providers (Martin, Hinds, and Felix, 1999; Parker and Gardner, 1992). Over the years the handwritten narrative has taken many forms in an attempt to effectively and efficiently document pertinent assessments and interventions, while allowing timely retrieval of pertinent data by other healthcare professionals. However, in today's healthcare environment, where inpatients are more acutely ill, staffing is short, and care is more complex, the documentation requirements and the need to have timely access to and reliable communication of patient care information to provide safe, quality care have continued to grow. Correspondingly, the pressure to streamline the collection, recording, and communication of data has been intense. Thus, clinicians are turning to point-of-care, online documentation systems to simplify these functions, increase the availability of data throughout the healthcare enterprise, and augment their practice with easy access to knowledge bases and decision support. The goals have not changed since the Institute of Medicine (IOM) report in 1991: records should be computer-based and used actively in the clinical process (IOM, 1991). But the mandate for today's automated tools is that they must be available and used as an integral part of the patient care delivery process, no matter the venue of care delivery—bedside, clinic exam room, or patient home—to enhance direct patient care (IOM 1997; Hughes 2000).

The past 10 years have seen a shift in reimbursement models, movement toward managed care emphasizing health maintenance and disease management, pressure for defining best practice using evidence-based research, and an increased need for patient-centered health records that integrate information from all care settings. Concurrently, empowered consumers are demanding better access to high-quality, affordable health care. This has caused leaders to see the work of nurses differently today (Porter-O'Grady 2001). Nursing's role in care coordination and management across the continuum is expanded, including the use of best-practice protocols, diagnosis-specific pathways, and decision support aids in the form of interactive alerts and online reference materials. None of this can be done without taking advantage of the impact of technology and the use of electronic patient records (Harsanyi et al. 2000; Valusek 2002).

As major efforts to adequately describe nursing's contribution in health care advance, extensive research has culminated in the development of numerous standardized languages. The previously independent standardized nursing language initiatives are evolving into an integrated, multidisciplinary, and even international effort aimed at accurately describing clinical practice and supporting decision-making. Some of these standardized nursing languages and concepts are becoming more commonly, although not universally, incorporated into nursing schools' curricula and course content, practice settings, and healthcare information systems.

Although knowledge work and intellectual capital have yet to garner ubiquitous recognition as the business of health care and of nursing, the increasing interest in gaining and maintaining market share through web portals and strategic information management provides unique opportunities for nursing (Sorrells-Jones and Weaver, 1999; Stewart 1997). Nurses are accepting the challenge to create innovative education, practice, and administration applications to meet consumer, student, and professional colleague needs through telehealth technologies.

These professional practice trends, along with patient safety initiatives described in the next section of this chapter, emphasize support of the care delivery process and not just accumulation of patient data. It has been documented that clinical errors are most often the byproduct of bad processes and not bad people (IOM 2000). This expectation has driven CIS requirements as well. For example, allergy checking during medication administration is no longer expected to be a passive presentation of a patient's current allergy list on the computer. Rather, computers should provide an automated process through the use of bar coding for positive patient identification and medication identification, with system evaluation and clinician notification of drug-allergy conflicts. This is summarized well by a quote from the Institute of Medicine's report: "A growing body of evidence supports the conclusion that various types of IT applications lead to improvements in safety, effectiveness, patient-centered-ness, timeliness, efficiency, and equity … nonetheless, IT has barely touched patient care" (IOM 2001).

Policy, Regulation, and Standards

Significant change has taken place within the last decade relative to policy, regulation, and standards development. Ten years ago, the primary concern of the healthcare system was cost rather than quality, as evidenced by widespread efforts to adopt and implement managed care. As the decade advanced, the need to achieve a competitive advantage in the market place became the top business issue. This focus soon gave way to an emphasis on deriving greater value from existing data. Today there is a renewed commitment to quality and the use of information technology to enhance patient safety. This section explores some of the external forces driving healthcare organizations to focus on implementing information technology applications that address quality and safety issues during the delivery of patient care.

Recent quality efforts include initiatives by the Agency for Healthcare Research and Quality (AHRQ) to fund patient safety research and the National Quality Forum's work developing standardized metrics that will accommodate valid quality comparisons across all healthcare organizations (HIMSS 2001). The Joint Commission on Accreditation of Healthcare Organizations (JCAHO) and the National Committee for Quality Assurance (NCQA) have been actively involved in patient safety initiatives as well (O'Leary 2001). The Institute of Medicine reports—*To Err is Human* (2000) and *Crossing the Quality Chasm* (2001)—have stimulated much public and private sector response, and have sharpened the focus on using technology to reduce medical errors (IOM 2000, 2001).

Perhaps the most striking outcome of these initiatives is the formal and informal pressure being applied to healthcare organizations for adopting technology as a primary means for enhancing patient safety. The Leapfrog Group, a coalition of corporations and employers that was recently joined by JCAHO, is using its combined power to compel provider and payer organizations to adopt initiatives that increase patient safety, such as computerized physician order entry (CPOE) systems and comparative data analysis tools. Together these employers flex enormous financial muscle in the healthcare system, spending over $52 billion on health benefits for more than 28 million people annually (Martinez 2002). Recent reports from this group have provided healthcare organizations with a guide for effective selection and implementation of such systems (Leapfrog 2001).

The Health Insurance Portability and Accountability Act (HIPAA) has captured the full attention of healthcare organizations. Specific provisions of this regulation, subtitled Administrative Simplification, establish standards for privacy and security of electronic health information, electronic data interchange (EDI) transactions and the use of unique health identifiers for each individual, employer, health plan, and provider. The focus on HIPAA compliance has displaced controlling costs and deriving more value from systems as the top business issue for healthcare information technology leaders (HIMSS 2002). Efforts to implement HIPAA-compliant systems are expected to impact information technology budgets for the next years (Coile 2001). Similarly, mandates for state and local data collection activities related to patient care outcomes and resource allocation assume that effective information systems are in place and operational. The flexibility of current systems is challenged to respond to changing methods of reporting to external agencies.

The International Classification of Nursing Practice (ICNP), Nursing Minimum Data Set (NMDS), Long Term Care Minimum Data Set, and other standards activities are influencing the development and implementation of information systems that support the automated exchange of clinical and financial data (Ozbolt et al. 2001). A convening body for standardization of languages within nursing is the Nursing Terminology Summit. Its mission is to promote and support the development, evaluation, and use of a reference terminology for nursing and its integration with healthcare applications and other healthcare terminological systems. The Summit functions as a think tank to resolve open questions at a high level, coordinate initiatives, and set directions for standards development to be carried out in other forums (Ozbolt 2002).

In response to rapid changes in nursing, computer and information sciences, emerging nursing informatics (NI) role specifications, and thinking within the specialty of informatics, the ANA convened a workgroup to review and revise *Scope of Practice for Nursing Informatics* and *Standards of Nursing Informatics*

(ANA 2001). This document expands on earlier work within nursing informatics, providing historical as well as state-of-the-science material for the specialty. This revision includes new sections on metastructures and concepts underpinning NI, human–computer interaction, and ergonomics concepts; the evolution of NI definitions; a definition, goal, and role specification for NI; informatics competencies and roles of informatics nurse specialists; ethics in nursing informatics; and revised standards of practice and professional performance.

Steady progress is also being made in the development of multidisciplinary language infrastructure and standards. The impact of the Systemized Nomenclature of Medicine (SNOMED) and standards—such as Health Level 7 (HL7) communication, American Society for Testing and Materials (ASTM), and International Organization for Standardization (ISO)—are far reaching. The Nursing Terminology Summit has provided significant input to both HL7 and SNOMED regarding extensions to ensure the ability to represent nursing adequately in the HL7 standards and the SNOMED Clinical Terms.

Utilization of existing standards such as HL7 and Digital Imaging and Communications in Medicine (DICOM) has enabled initiatives such as Integrating the Healthcare Enterprise (IHE), whose technical framework provides an implementation to successfully link the radiology systems environment, to begin to deliver on the promise of true cross-system integration (Wirsz 2001).

The availability of national and international standards, combined with policy, regulatory, and economic forces, result in a scenario that drives technology adoption from virtually all perspectives. To impact the quality of care and improve patient safety, technology must support process-driven systems that provide real-time information to clinicians during the delivery of patient care, and not just retrospective data analysis or performance reporting.

Technology

Leading the evolution of technology is the development of enabling technologies that support current healthcare delivery processes. In the hardware category, the availability of wireless devices, the impact of the Internet and satellite technology, and disk space that was hardly imagined 10 years ago dramatically broadens the capability of supporting applications that meet the needs of nurses and other clinicians. The mouse/browser/hyperlink paradigm facilitates the availability of web-enabled transactions and access to knowledge resources and other types of information for both providers and patients within the context of the clinical encounter. A more secure computing environment is supported by the use of encryption, digital certificates, and public key infrastructure (PKI) technologies.

Increasing numbers of devices provide the technological platform for the implementation of applications that seamlessly support workflow and just-in-time information gathering, not only for clinicians, but also for healthcare consumers. Tools such as personal digital assistants (PDAs), cellular phones with personal computing capability, bedside devices, and hand-held computers using wireless technologies can accommodate remote monitoring and surveillance in traditional and telehealth settings. Recent HIMSS Annual Leadership Surveys reflect this trend as respondents identify wireless information appliances as the most important technology of the future (HIMSS 2002). Newer mobile computing applications provide clinicians with the ability to handle point-of-care activities including medical referencing, clinical documentation, alert messaging, and prescription writing, as well as administrative tasks such as charge capture and general communications (Turisco and Case 2001). This further enables the increased reliance on healthcare services within diverse ambulatory settings.

A key technological change is the broadened understanding and use of knowledge representation methodologies and tools in healthcare informatics that support semantic and syntactic models. Unified Modeling Language (UML), Extensible Markup Language (XML), conceptual graphs, and other representation methodologies are more widely used. Additionally, efforts are underway to incorporate legacy coding schemas into current semantic models. This has resulted in a framework that provides the infrastructure for collection, processing, storage, and exchange of standardized clinical data and information within and between clinical information systems.

Another critical evolving technology is object-oriented software engineering. The growing understanding of the use of this technology in the development of clinical applications yields integrated, scalable applications. Incorporation of object orientation into all phases of the software development lifecycle is increasingly recognized as the means for developing and implementing true software solutions. Particularly significant is the ability of object modeling to represent the clinical domain in a way that can be understood, interpreted, and used in requirements documents for programming of clinical software. Object models provide a communication mechanism between clinical domain experts and software engineers, removing one of the key barriers (Detmer and Shortliffe 1995).

The arrival of the Internet offers the opportunity to fundamentally reinvent medicine and healthcare delivery. The e-health era is nothing less than the digital transformation of the practice of medicine and of the business aspects of the health industry (Coile 2002). However, in spite of its seeming promise, Wall Street values for e-health companies have gone from boom to bust. Analysts attribute the rapid collapse of the e-health sector to the slow pace of healthcare providers' adoption of new technology (Coile 2002). Although the promise of e-health has not been realized, the maintenance of electronic personal health records has become an option for the healthcare consumer. Smart card technology is available but not yet in widespread circulation. As healthcare organizations struggle to incorporate e-health strategies, the consumer is challenged to become a partner in their care and to make use of the information technology that provides access to their lifetime health record.

Return on investment for information technology is being realized with evidence that the most wired healthcare organizations have better control of expenses, higher productivity, and more efficient utilization management (Solovy 2001). In spite of these findings, it is noteworthy that not all of these technological advances have been truly leveraged by healthcare providers, information systems developers, and vendors. However, their increasing availability significantly broadens the technological landscape upon which clinical applications that support workflow during the care delivery process can be based.

Information Systems

Information systems are prevalent in healthcare organizations today, and their focus is beginning to move beyond the financial impetus of years past. The number and type of applications are striking, and current systems include specialized features and functions for all areas of professional practice. Clinical information systems with applications to support human decision-making and outcomes analysis are slowly being integrated into practice. Respondents to recent HIMSS surveys (2002) identified clinical systems as the most important applications for the next 2 years. Applications abound for specialties—such as critical care, community health, ambulatory care, and nursing administration—and provide much-needed technology to support the work of nurses. Expert systems are available that include a knowledge base brimming with facts along with an inference engine designed to replicate the reasoning and decision-making of clinical experts (McHugh 2001). Pattern recognition and problem solving are important aspects of artificial intelligence systems. These systems can also track the accuracy of their predictions and alter their own decision-making rules based on new knowledge that is generated. Natural language systems are emerging that can understand and process commands given in the user's own natural, spoken language (McHugh 2001). These systems are designed to recognize and process human speech and/or handwriting.

The use of clinical decision support systems to enhance clinical performance and the parallel migration toward utilizing best-practice models and evidence-based practice demonstrate the impact that is being realized from the improvement in clinical systems. The convergence of systems that support disease management, quality improvement, and clinical efficiency has demonstrated the impact of information technology on the quality of patient care (HIMSS 2001). The benefits of CPOE and the use of bar code technology to improve patient safety have been widely recognized although few institutions have successfully installed these systems (Ahmad et al. 2002). The Veterans Health Administration is a notable exception, demonstrating an overall 75% decrease in medication errors after system-wide implementation of Bar Code Medication Administration (BCMA) software (Johnson et al. 2002).

The increased emphasis on evidence-based practice, which focuses on accessing, critically analyzing, and applying evidence to practice can be supported with embedded rules and communications links in information systems (Bakken 2001). Prompts and alerts, defined clinical pathways for care delivery, and order templates provide feedback on the accuracy and relevance of diagnostic and treatment strategies (Andolina 2000). Access to references and scientific literature combine with statistical analysis and graphics tools to support decision-making. With "write once and use many times" capability, nursing and other professions can use the same data, information, and knowledge for diverse purposes as part of the delivery of evidence-based practice. However, a number of barriers still remain, including the rapid development of healthcare knowledge, inconsistent ability to access to information at the point of care, and increased patient complexity (Bakken 2001).

With recent advances in computer software, nurse executives use management information systems to perform such functions as fiscal and human resource management, strategic planning, policy formulation, and workload measurement (Shamian and Hannah 2000). Nurse executives acknowledge the value of utilizing computing power to manage data and information to demonstrate administrative leadership. As the core business of health care continues to expand beyond the walls of the hospital, management information systems provide the capability of incorporating information from a patient's multiple episodes of care. Use of the Nursing Management Minimum Data Set (NMMDS) will provide the standardization needed to make comparisons about care effectiveness within and across healthcare institutions (Huber, Schumacher, and Delaney 1997); however, widespread implementation of the NMMDS remains unrealized.

Although information systems and clinical applications have proliferated, the growing number of healthcare systems and networks represent a significant challenge for connecting them in a seamless web of coordinated care (Coile 2002). Integrated systems are available from single vendors, but cross-vendor integration has not been realized. Software applications using communication standards such as HL7 and DICOM are being implemented with mixed success. A decade-long study of integration in leading integrated delivery networks (IDN) across the nation reports that information systems continue to be inadequate in the critical function of physician and clinical integration (Shortell et al. 2000). Study authors encourage IDNs of the future to expand the focus of their information systems from business processes to clinical care and quality management. In summary, although an increasing number and variety of clinical information systems are available, widespread adoption of these technologies has not been realized.

Human Factors

Human factors, the fifth category, encompass the broad area of effective interaction between human beings and computers. Human factors engineering provides both a body of knowledge about the human abilities, limitations, and characteristics that are relevant to design, and the processes, tools, and techniques for applying that knowledge during the design process (Gosbee and Gardner-Bonneau 1998). This body of knowledge applies to the physical interface between the user and the system as well as the behavioral aspects, including information about sensation and perception, human information processing, memory, attention, and decision-making as they affect human performance. The design of the user interface has long been a topic of interest. However, a focus on quick technological solutions has often resulted in problems in the daily use of applications, particularly those applications that attempt to automate complex processes.

In the past five years, a growing appreciation of the complexity of human–computer interaction (HCI), as well as a better understanding of reasoning and decision making processes has emerged. Key developments in the field of HCI include recognition of the importance of iterative evaluation of user interfaces during the design process. Combining iterative design processes with the emerging field of usability engineering results in development approaches that include early and rapid prototyping. Usability concepts, which refer to the capacity of the system to allow users to carry out their tasks safely and effectively, are being incorporated into healthcare systems and operations (Staggers 2000). Usability engineering and testing involve formalized methods to evaluate and improve the usability of systems. In the field of healthcare informatics, usability has historically been a key deterrent to the adoption of clinical information systems (Gosbee and Gardner-Bonneau 1998). The growing understanding of iterative design and usability testing as means to increase the human–computer interaction is a marked change, and improvement, in the development of clinical information systems.

Other influences and factors must also be considered in the discussion of human factors. Individual access to and familiarity with personal computing resources may create unrealistic expectations in the HIS environment. Complex software applications and networks do not respond as readily as a personal computer-based environment. Similarly, expectations about web access for business purposes may not match personal use at home because of security and resource limitations. Resistance to learning, fear of standardization, and distrust of vendors also impact the acceptance of new technology.

Current systems can accommodate a variety of data capture methods that are close to the time and source of creation. Bar code readers, touch screen capability, speech recognition, hand-held or notebook devices, and remote, wireless computing options enhance the accuracy and efficiency of data entry while minimizing the amount of human interaction that is necessary. User interface characteristics that include consistent terminology, simple, clear and frequent exits, feedback and instructions, and ease of use contribute to system acceptance (Douglas 2001). The intuitive appearance and user friendliness of help features enhance the effectiveness of human–computer interactions. Great strides have been made in understanding the HCI of clinicians. This knowledge, if used to influence the design of devices and applications that support the delivery of patient care, will contribute to broader acceptance by clinicians.

Technology Adoption

Health care is a complex and information-intensive industry. Collaborative practice agreements have established new business models. Mergers, acquisitions, and divestitures in enterprise organizations characterize today's environment. The resulting clinical and financial reporting requirements, development of composite pharmaceutical formularies and data dictionaries, and diverse system integration initiatives similarly reflect this increasing complexity and necessary commitment to electronic and integrated delivery networks.

Increasing reliance on integrated information system technologies and instant access in all other aspects of life spills over into health care. There is near-universal use of automatic teller machines (ATMs) and bar coded grocery store checkout. Electronic funds transfer for payroll, social security, credit card transactions, electronic tax filing, and online electronic commerce are quickly becoming the norm. Computer skills development in preschool and elementary educational curricula, as well as exposure to online catalogs of library journals and other resources, reinforce the expectations of technology-astute clinicians and consumers for similar resources in the healthcare environment.

Historically, the predominant philosophy for the adoption and use of technology has been grounded in the mindset that technology, as it evolves and advances, is the solution to a variety of business, professional, and personal problems. For over 20 years, technology and automation have been heralded as the means by which complex problems are solved. A key assumption is the notion that users must adopt technology as presented, even though it does not really solve these problems in an elegant way. To the contrary, adopting technology may even complicate the situation. For example, electronic calendaring applications are basically good ideas, but are not necessarily easy to learn or use. Nonetheless, users have adopted such applications along with all of their limitations because these tools are seen to be advantageous over paper calendars—one chooses to pay the price of more complex appointment entry to reap the benefit of access and simplified meeting planning.

Policy, legislative, economic, and cultural factors strongly and fundamentally support technology adoption in all aspects of life, whether or not that technology provides solutions. A dependence on and expectation that automation is the primary means to improve processes has evolved in business, commercial, communication, and personal interaction environments. Automated functionality is a fundamental part of the daily experience of all individuals, again regardless of whether it provides a solution to any particular problem. Critical to this pervasive perspective is the appreciation that technology has indeed provided many significant solutions to business, communication, and personal issues. However, the more complex of these often have not been solved. And it is in this category that the business and communication processes of clinical care reside.

Integrating technology into a complex clinical workflow is not easy—defining the application to be used, on what kind of device, and how the clinician and/or patient will interact with it requires detailed analysis. Clinicians are quick to complain about application design, but often cannot find the time to assist in the design up front. Adoption of clinical applications usually requires providers to change workflow patterns and routines to accommodate the system. The process of finding a computer, logging on, selecting a patient, choosing a function, and then completing the entry can be tedious (Chan 2002). Even hand-held or other remote devices are found to have their shortcomings. Often the clinician who pays the price by collecting the data and entering it into the computer may not be the one who reaps the benefit by accessing the data later. All of these aspects contribute to the difficulty with adoption of technology during clinical application implementation, despite the fact that these same clinicians have embraced technology for numerous other processes in their lives.

Finally, the increased availability of information must be considered in this discussion. Ten years ago, Microsoft Windows was in development and very few healthcare consumers owned computers. Today, overall adoption of technology in society has resulted in an increasing number of Americans using the Internet and e-mail, with a significant increase in access to information by healthcare consumers (Lewis 1999). According to an April 2002 Harris Poll, of the 137 million Americans who surf the Internet, more than 60% use it as a resource for health advice. This number increased approximately 5% from 2001 (Landro 2002). Information that was previously the purview of the clinician is now accessible to everyone at the touch on a keyboard or click of a mouse. A key impact of this increased access is a shift in the power relationships of patients, providers, and insurers in the e-health environment. Healthcare consumers, previously the unempowered in these relationships, now frequently come to the healthcare encounter with more clinical information than the provider who will prescribe their care (Lewis 1999; Staggers, Thompson, and Snyder-Halpern 2001). The impact of this realignment of power, based on information, is increasingly evident. Healthcare providers, healthcare organizations, and HIS vendors systems are scrambling to provide the means to not only be the source of healthcare information for consumers, but also to ensure that healthcare organizations and providers have adequate information to deal effectively with their well-informed clients (Lewis and Friedman 2000).

System Utilization

A logical and often repeated statement in healthcare computing is that applications must be easy for clinicians to use. However, what constitutes ease of use is seldom documented (Staggers 2000). This chapter addressed this complex issue by describing the essentials of system utilization: type of information system, quality of human–computer interaction, technology used and adopted, and the degree of system integration within the nursing practice process model. A discussion of the policy, regulation, and standards that underpin utilization was also presented.

Key transitions have taken place in each of the categories over the past decade, and these changes lay the groundwork for defining future systems that support the work of nurses. Significant progress has been made in understanding the characteristics necessary for successful clinical system implementation in this fourth phase, where implementation is driven by the ease with which the technology integrates into the care process workflow. If the technology is easy to use, integrates well into existing workflow, and benefits nursing, it will be used. However, if the balance of these factors is tipped in alternative ways, then system utilization may be impacted.

References

Ahmad, A., P. Teater, T. D. Bentley, L. Kuehn, R. R. Kumar, A. Thomas, and H. S. Mekhjian. 2002. Key attributes of a successful physician order entry system implementation in a multi-hospital environment. *Journal of the American Medical Informatics Association* 9(1): 16–24.

American Nurses Association (ANA). 2001. *Scope and Standards of Informatics Nursing Practice.* Washington, DC: American Nurses Publishing.

Andolina, K. M. 2000. The automation of clinical pathways. In *Nursing Informatics: Where Caring and Technology Meet*, edited by M. J. Ball, J. Hannah, S. K. Newbold, and J. V. Douglas. New York: Springer.

Bakken, S. 2001. Informatics in support of evidence-based practice. *Journal of the American Medical Informatics Association* 8(3): 199–201.

Chan, W. 2002. Increasing the success of physician order entry through human factors engineering. *Journal of Healthcare Information Management* 16(1): 71–79.

Coile, R. 2001. *HIMSS HIT Forecast: 2002–2006: Health Information Technology in the New Millennium.* Chicago: Healthcare Information and Management Systems Society.

———. 2002. *The Paperless Hospital: Healthcare in a Digital Age.* Chicago: Foundation of the American College of Healthcare Executives.

Detmer, W. M., and E. H. Shortliffe. 2002. A model of clinical query management that supports integration of biomedical information over the World Wide Web. Section on Medical Informatics: Stanford University School of Medicine. 1995 [cited 2002]. Available from URL: http://smi-web.stanford.edu/pubs/SMI_Reports/SMI-95-0577.pdf.

Douglas, M. 2001. Implementing and upgrading clinical information systems. In *Essentials of Computers for Nurses: Informatics for the New Millennium*, edited by V. K. Saba, and K. McCormick. New York: McGraw-Hill.

Gosbee, J., and D. Gardner-Bonneau. 1998. The human factor. *Healthcare Informatics* 15(2): 141–143.

Harsanyi, B. E., K. C. Allan, J. Anderson, C. Valo, J. M. Fitzpatrick, E. A. Schofield, S. Benjamiin, and B. W. Simundza. 2000. Healthcare information systems. In *Nursing Informatics: Where Caring and Technology Meet*, edited by M. J. Ball, K. J. Hannah, S. K. Newbold, and J. V. Douglas. New York: Springer.

Healthcare Information and Management Systems Society (HIMSS). 2001. *The Healthcare IT Environment: Strategies for Providers and Vendors.* Chicago: HIMSS.

———. 2002. *Annual HIMSS/Hewlett Packard Leadership Survey.* Chicago: HIMSS.

Huber, D., L. Schumacher, and C. Delaney. 1997. Nursing management minimum data set (NMMDS). *Journal of Nursing Administration* 27(4): 42–48.

Hughes, S. J. 2000. Point-of-care information systems: State of the art. In *Nursing Informatics: Where Caring and Technology Meet*, edited by M. J. Ball, K. J. Hannah, S. K. Newbold, and J. V. Douglas. New York: Springer.

IOM (Institute of Medicine). 1991. *The Computer-based Patient Record: An Essential Technology for Change.* (Authors R. Dick and E. Steen). Washington, DC: Institute of Medicine.

————. 1997. *The Computer-Based Patient Record: An Essential Technology for Healthcare, Revised Edition.* (R. S. Dick, E. B. Steen, and D. E. Detmer, eds.) Washington, DC: National Academy Press.

————. 2001. *Crossing the Quality Chasm.* Committee on Quality of Health Care in America, Washington, DC: National Academy Press.

Johnson, C. L., R. A. Carlson, C. L. Tucker, and C. Willette. 2002. Using BCMA software to improve patient safety in Veterans Administration medical centers. *Journal of Healthcare Information Management* 16(1): 46–51.

Landro, L. 2002. The informed patient: if doctors prescribe information, will patients pay or surf Web? *The Wall Street Journal* 2002 (April 25 2002; page D4). Available also from URL: http://online.wsj.com/ (for subscribers).

Leapfrog (Leapfrog Group and First Consulting Group). 2001. *Overview of the Leapfrog Group Evaluation Tool for Computerized Physician Order Entry.* December 2001. First Consulting Group. Also available from URL: http://www.leapfroggroup.org/ under *CPOE Reports.*

Lewis, D. 1999. Computer-based approaches to patient education: a review of the literature. *Journal of the American Medical Informatics Association* 6(4): 272–282.

Lewis, D., and C. Friedman. 2000. Consumer health informatics. In *Nursing Informatics: Where Caring and Technology Meet*, edited by M. J. Ball, K. J. Hannah, S. K. Hannah and J. V. Douglas. New York: Springer.

Martin, A., C. Hinds, and M. Felix. 1999. Documentation practices of nurses in long-term care. *Journal of Clinical Nursing* 8(3): 345–352.

Martinez, B. 2002. Employers group's strategy aims to save lives, money by reducing medical errors. *The Wall Street Journal*, January 17. Available from URL: http://online.wsj.com/ (for subscribers).

McHugh, M. 2001. Computer Systems. In *Essentials of Computers for Nurses: Informatics for the New Millennium,* 3rd ed., edited by V. K. Saba and K. McCormick. New York: McGraw-Hill.

O'Leary, D. 2001. *Statement of the Joint Commission on Accreditation of Healthcare Organizations before the U.S. Senate and the Subcommittee on Labor, Health and Human Services and Education of the Senate Committee on Appropriations, February 22, 2001.* Joint Commission on Accreditation of Healthcare Operations 2001 [cited 2002]. Available from URL: http://www.jcaho.org/.

Ozbolt, J. 2002. Mission of the Terminology Summit. Paper read at *Nursing Terminology Summit Conference* 2002, June 27–30, 2002, at Vanderbilt University, Nashville, Tenn.

Ozbolt, J., I. Abraham, and S. Schultz II. 1990. Nursing information systems. In *Medical Informatics: Computer Applications in Healthcare*, edited by E. Shortliffe, and L. Perrault. Reading, MA: Addison-Wesley.

Ozbolt, J., I. Androwich, S. Bakken, P. Button, N. Hardiker, C. Mead, J. Warren, and C. Zingo. 2001. *The Nursing Terminology Summit Conference 2001: Resolving ambiguities at the intersections of conceptual structures.* S-28 Panel at the 2001 Symposium of the American Medical Informatics Association. (November 3–7, 2001.) Washington, DC: AMIA.

Parker, J., and G. Gardner. 1992. The silence and silencing of the nurses voice: A reading of patient progress notes. *The Australian Journal of Advanced Nursing* 9(3): 3–8.

Porter-O'Grady, T. 2001. Into the new age: The call for a new construct for nursing. *Geriatric Nursing* 22(1): 12–15.

Shamian, J., and K. J. Hannah. 2000. Management information systems for the nurse executive. In *Nursing Informatics: Where Caring and Technology Meet*, edited by M. J. Ball, K. J. Hannah, S. K. Newbold, and J. V. Douglas. New York: Springer.

Shortell, S. M., R. R. Gillies, D. A. Anderson, K. M. Erickson, and J. B. Mitchell. 2000. *Remaking Health Care in America: The Evolution of Organized Delivery Systems,* 2nd ed. San Francisco: Jossey-Bass.

Solovy, A. 2001. The Big Payback. 2001 survey shows a healthy return on investment for info tech. *Hospitals and Health Networks* 75(7): 40–50.

Sorrells-Jones, J., and D. Weaver. 1999. Knowledge workers and knowledge-intense organizations. Part 1: A promising framework for nursing and healthcare. *Journal of Nursing Administration* 19(7/8): 12–18.

Staggers, N. 2000. Usability concepts and clinical computing. In *Nursing Informatics: Where Caring and Technology Meet*, edited by M. J. Ball, K. J. Hannah, S. K. Newbold, and J. V. Douglas. New York: Springer.

Stagggers, N., C. B. Thompson, and R. Snyder-Halpern. 2001. History and trends in clinical information systems in the United States. *Journal of Nursing Scholarship* 33(1): 75–81.

Stewart, T. A. 1997. *Intellectual Capital*. New York: Doubleday/Currency.

Turisco, F., and J. Case. 2001. *Wireless and Mobile Computing* [World Wide Web]. California Healthcare Foundation 2001 [cited October 2001]. Available from URL: http://www.ehealth.chcf.org.

Valusek, J. R. 2002. Decision support: A paradigm addition for patient safety. *Journal of Healthcare Information Management* 16(1): 34–39.

Wirsz, N. 2001. IHE: Future directions. In *Integrating the Healthcare Enterprise*, edited by P. R. Vegoda. Chicago: HIMSS.

Implications | 4

The purpose of this chapter is to discuss the implications of what the authors have learned regarding the status of clinical information systems (CISs) 10 years ago and now. Chapters 2 and 3, the authors documented in great detail the environment and status of clinical information systems. This provides a baseline against which the authors have described our current reality in the context of the organizing framework of the monograph.

A Major Conceptual Shift

This reality is perhaps most graphically demonstrated in the striking contrast between the recommendations of the Institute of Medicine in 1991 (*The Computer-Based Patient Record: An Essential Technology for Health Care*) and a decade later in 2001 in *Crossing the Quality Chasm: A New Health System for the 21st Century* (IOM 2001; IOM 1991). The 1991 recommendations included a broad, sweeping, comprehensive approach at the core of which was the recommendation to adopt the computerized patient record (CPR) as the standard for medical records. This recommendation described the ideal medical record as having 180 key features in 12 categories. The scope of the recommended CPR was ambitious because it included so many perspectives, and so many stakeholders. Perhaps most important to this discussion, it also included multiple complexities—terminologies, networks, security, data versus documents, integration, and required significant organizational change. Today the 180 characteristics are variably present in available systems and those that are present are variably implemented. In addition, due in part to multiple false starts and restarts, the anticipated return on investment (ROI) of the adoption of the CPR both in dollars and patients outcomes has not been uniformly achieved.

The IOM recommendations in *Crossing the Quality Chasm* (IOM 2001) are very different from those made in 1991. First, the 2001 recommendations focus on information technology as a *means* versus an end in itself.

A fully electronic medical record, including all types of patient information, is not needed to achieve many, if not most, of the benefits of automated clinical data. The committee believes information technology must play a central role in the redesign of the healthcare system if a substantial improvement in quality is to be achieved over the coming decade. Automation of clinical, financial, and administrative transactions is essential to improving quality, preventing errors, enhancing consumer confidence in the health system, and improving quality (p. 16).

However, the real focus of the IOM in 2001 is not the electronic medical record; rather it is a focus on care that is safe, effective, patient-centered, timely, efficient, and equitable. Information technology is positioned as a critical tool to be used in redesigned systems of care that will achieve the type of care described. Therefore, the recommendations related to information technology are in the overall context of quality.

If we want safer, higher quality care, we will need to have redesigned systems of care, including use of information technology, to support clinical and administrative processes (IOM 2001, p. 4).

As one considers the marked changes in perspective of the two IOM reports, a major shift in the conceptualization of the role and scope of the electronic medical record is clear. This shift reinforces the conceptual framework of this monograph regarding the role of information systems in supporting not only the capture and management of data, but also redesigned workflow processes. Additionally, the electronic medical record provides the means to capture data and information about professional practice. This shift in the role and scope of the electronic medical record confirms the complexity involved in achieving full automation of the work processes and content that are represented. In retrospect, thinking in the early 1990s failed to acknowledge that when automating a record of patient care, one needs to not only capture data, but also understand and represent the underlying processes involved in that care.

Constraints

A number of constraints have impeded progress in the development and implementation of systems that truly support workflow and capture critical clinical data. These constraints have existed in relation to all of the major concepts in our framework—professional practice process understanding; policy, regulation and standards; technology; information systems; human factors; technology adoption; and system utilization. However, significant changes and progress have taken place in the last decade related to these constraints.

For example, we have made important progress in professional nursing practice process understanding by not only defining nursing in vocabularies, but also by recognizing the need to develop the necessary infrastructure so that these languages can be integrated in information systems. In the policy arena, dramatic and groundbreaking initiatives have resulted in a very different paradigm for quality and systems in health care that defines information systems as a means, not an end in themselves. This shift positions nursing and nursing informaticists to leverage the changes in technology and technology adoption as never before. Changes in technology—both in enabling technologies and standardized knowledge representation and modeling methodologies—are also available for use and integration. Last, the healthcare industry has begun to recognize and address the implementation of human factors in the design of the user interface, as well as the implementation and change management processes.

So, it is fascinating to find that we are still struggling to get these information systems designed and implemented. The authors' perspective is that in our current reality, the paradigm that has emerged provides a very positive and encouraging framework for real progress in the near future. The described changes of the past 10 years are truly significant—they represent a fundamental shift in conceptualizing CISs as means versus ends and a shift from data-driven to data and workflow-driven systems. Inherent in this shift is an appreciation of the deep complexity involved in designing systems to support clinical workflow and content; a shift in the motivation for developing and implementing clinical systems based on policy and standards changes; a shift in society's positioning of information technology in daily life; and, perhaps most important, a shift in the appreciation of key methodologies to develop software that adequately addresses the inherent complexity. It is notable and positive that all of these changes have taken place, providing the platform for launching efforts to develop and implement systems that meet the expectations set forth more than 10 years ago.

Implications

In the context of the significant paradigm shift, newly appreciated complexity and insight into the constraints that have limited our ability to exploit information technology, informatics knowledge, and methods, what are the implications?

Implementing Our Knowledge and Learnings

We are not implementing either what we know or what we have learned. Over the past 10 years, there have been multiple information systems developed and many information systems projects implemented in health care and other industries. These projects have included work related to user-centered design, workflow analysis, and technology adoption models. In addition, there has been significant research completed in the areas of clinical processes, system implementation, and organizational change. The combined knowledge from this research and experience is rich with insights and specific implications for what needs to be done, as well as how to do it with increased likelihood of success. However, we are not adequately leveraging this knowledge in our current work.

Systems developed by vendors do not meet the needs and expectations of organizations. The systems do not reflect integration of the findings of research and experience. Nor do the implementation strategies in organizations reflect these learnings and research. There continues to be a knowledge-transfer gap between what is learned in academic research and what is available in the vendor/supplier marketplace. Even when the gap is identified, the time to market for the new innovation is simply too long. This gap, and the delay in getting to market, end up being significant to clinical system projects. Hence, many systems implemented today have little support of workflow or decision-making, and continue to be primarily data-driven and not workflow- or knowledge-driven. Overall, there appears to be an interesting pattern of making the same mistakes over and over in our clinical systems' projects. We can no longer afford to invest time, energy, and dollars in system development and implementation that does not take into account what we have learned multiple times.

Learning New Skills and Approaches

We must learn some new skills and approaches. Throughout this monograph, the topics of business modeling, complex project management, team leadership and participation, communication and change management have been mentioned in the context of the complexity of development and implementation of clinical systems. It is probably inaccurate to describe any of these as new skills and approaches. Some of them, particularly business modeling, are newer to health care. However, similar to the integration of knowledge from research and experience, we have not systematically incorporated these skills and approaches in our educational programs or in our work in either provider or vendor organizations. Nursing informatics is still a very young and developing discipline. There are relatively few seasoned nurse informaticians who truly understand and can lead the implementation with the skills and approaches described here. As a result of this lack of the understanding and systematic use of these methodologies, providers, vendors, and organizations struggle to define executable requirements and to implement systems that will indeed support the type of care described in *Crossing the Quality Chasm*.

Redesigning Aspects of Our Systems

We must redesign certain aspects of our systems. This is a particularly important implication. As discussed, we are entering a fourth phase of clinical information systems reflecting our understanding on how to build systems that not only capture and manage data, but that also meaningfully support improved workflow and care based on knowledge. The IOM, in *Crossing the Quality Chasm*, describes the critical care processes that are needed in the healthcare system (IOM 2001):

- Care based on continuous healing relationships.
- Customization based on patient needs and values.
- The patient as the source of control, shared knowledge, and the free flow of information.
- Evidence-based decision-making, with safety as a system priority.
- Anticipation of needs, and cooperation of clinicians.

These care processes—sounding somewhat like motherhood-and-apple-pie—represent astounding complexity, and are not easy to achieve in our information systems. It is only through methodical and painstaking use of standards and methodologies that we will be able to describe and represent these processes in such a way that we can build systems to support them.

Summary

As the authors review these implications, it appears that there is still a missing ingredient, an aspect not yet addressed thoroughly in this monograph. Simply stated, we must recognize that what we have been doing is not working. For in the face of all that has been developed, learned, researched, and defined as policy, we continue to struggle to develop and implement systems that meet even minimal expectations of the true potential of information systems to not only make care delivery more efficient, but to transform it.

A critical aspect of this hard-to-face reality is that we appear to lack openness to change. Christensen, Bohmer and Kenagy, in the *Harvard Business Review*, stated that "Health care may be the most entrenched, change-averse industry in the United States. The innovations that will eventually turn us around are ready, in some cases—but they can't find backers" (Christensen, Bohmer, and Kenagy 2000). These authors further state that in the face of this resistance to change, the only hope for the US healthcare industry is openness to what they describe as "disruptive innovation"—innovation that is characterized by disruptive technologies and business models that, although they may threaten the status quo, are the means to raise the overall quality of care. In nursing, we have had a strong history of considering ourselves *not* to be resistant—but rather to be harbingers of innovation and change. However, in the clinical systems arena, if not in other areas, there is an acute need for serious soul searching and self-examination around our openness to giving up old models and behaviors, old frameworks of reality, and to embrace learning new methodologies and skills.

The challenge for nursing educators, administrators, practitioners, researchers, and informaticists resides in the willingness to adopt new models of behavior, assuming leadership that is based on what we have learned through experience and research. Our challenge is to give up the "nursing" perspective and become true team members with other clinicians as well as with software developers and vendors, while appropriately describing and supporting nursing's unique contributions. Additionally we must apply newfound skills in modeling and designing systems. All of this implies the need for strong leadership that can demonstrate the application of the tools, policies, research, methods, and experience to embrace and build on the true changes of the past 10 years. This implies a need for true leadership, which is often a lonely and uncomfortable position.

As we define a vision for clinical information systems for the next generation, it is paramount that we keep these implications in mind. The revisiting of the principles and guidelines for clinical information systems, the purpose of this monograph, will only result in truly effective change if it is based on the application of our learnings and growth. It is not sufficient to work harder doing the same things; rather, we must truly function in a new paradigm. In Chapter 5, the authors describe a vision for clinical systems in this new paradigm and make specific recommendations to achieve the vision.

References

Christensen, C. M., R. Bohmer, and J. Kenagy. 2000. Will disruptive innovations cure health care? *Harvard Business Review* September-October: 102–110.

IOM (Institute of Medicine). 1991. (Authors: R. Dick and E. Steen.) *The Computer-based Patient Record: An Essential Technology for Change*. Washington, DC: Institute of Medicine.

————. 2001. Committee on Quality of Health Care in America. *Crossing the Quality Chasm*. Washington, DC: National Academy Press.

Vision & Recommendations 5

The purpose of this monograph is to revisit the principles and guidelines for clinical information systems (CISs) to support nursing practice in light of the events, learnings, and other forces of the past 10 years. Based on the analysis described in Chapters 2 and 3, the principles and guidelines described in the *Next-Generation* monograph (Zielstorff, Hudgings, and Grobe 1993) continue to be valid; many of the key assumptions described still apply. And there is no question that many if not all of the functional requirements outlined in the monograph are still required (see Appendix A).

However, it also appears that the functionality of a new generation of clinical information systems must extend beyond meeting basic data and information needs to support professional nursing practice. It is also clear that the processes for developing, implementing, and using systems must change. Therefore, the principles and guidelines for clinical information systems to support nursing practice must be broadened. Both a vision and an organizing framework are needed that reflect the conceptual shift in thinking about systems as an end to systems as tools, tools that support the processes of care delivery and knowledge management. Presentation of this new vision and discussion of a new organizing framework to guide the development, implementation, and use of clinical information systems follows. The recommendations to achieve the vision and key strategies for implementation will guide CIS development, implementation, and use.

Vision

In the vision of the future, nurses in all domains of professional nursing practice have the data, information, and knowledge resources to inform and complete their work. Nursing education and practice continue to change as a result of a closed feedback loop between practice and practice process understanding. Data, information, and knowledge are available and are used. Computers are ubiquitous. Fundamental process change has occurred, thereby creating measurable differences in nursing practice compared to the past. These processes improve individual healthcare encounters at the moment of the encounter and provide feedback for subsequent, more in-depth review. Thus, nursing practice reflects a dual purpose—the one-to-one clinical encounter of the individual nurse with a patient and the aggregation of information for analysis and iterative generation of knowledge to transform practice.

Knowledge informs every patient encounter and generates new knowledge for future patient encounters so that the next encounter is improved. Each clinician welcomes and embraces knowledge, expects the healthcare system and the information system to provide knowledge resources, and integrates and acts on that available knowledge in practice. Patients expect and even demand informed healthcare clinicians who accept, support, and value their active individual participation in acquiring shared knowledge and clinical decision-making.

Clinical information systems evolve, providing data, information, and knowledge contributing to constant, iterative change in nursing practice, workflows, and healthcare quality. Clinician use of systems is integrated into practice and has become an expectation of patients, who understand the safety and quality implications of CIS use.

Innovation is a cultural norm in nursing and health care. Nurses willingly leave behind current ways of working and embrace a better way. The information system supports and enables change, serving as a transforming and powerful tool that leverages what is in the literature, other databases, policies, and guidelines, combined with local data, information, and knowledge into every encounter.

The healthcare environment and information systems allow clinicians to comfortably say, "I don't know, but I can easily find out." The clinicians know what they do not know and trust the system to give them needed information and access to knowledge, policy, and standards resources to resolve the deficits. They expect an information system to be pervasive, trustworthy, and useful. Clinicians are uncomfortable when they must practice without an available information system.

The system's human-machine interaction seems natural, integrates into the workflow, and is worthy of trust, becoming a common tool that is part of the daily routine, available when needed—just like today's stethoscope. Compatible technologies ensure that information is integrated and universal. For example, if an email includes an embedded message or image, selecting the link immediately accesses that content.

In 1990, it was possible to envision the technology and expect it to come to fruition. In 2002, the technology exists, but the vision of how to use that technology to transform health care is, as yet, unrealized.

New Organizing Framework

To formulate meaningful recommendations to achieve the vision, it is helpful to revisit the organizing framework of this monograph. In the preceding chapters, we used an organizing framework to develop an understanding of:

- The original recommendations from the *Next-Generation* monograph (Zielstorff, Hudgings, and Grobe 1993) and the Institute of Medicine report on the computer-based patient record (IOM 1991).

- Past challenges that hampered progress in clinical information systems.
- Contemporary factors that influence information system development and implementation.
- Impediments preventing achievement of the full set of recommendations in the *Next-Generation* monograph.
- What is and is not important for CIS development.
- What remains to be done.

The original framework (see Figure 1-1, p. 4) delineates a set of hierarchical concepts that illustrate the complex factors involved in systems and the relationships of those concepts. An analysis of these factors resulted in the identification of those aspects of the framework that have been deemphasized in systems development to date. The concept of professional nursing practice process understanding has not driven the definition of functional requirements for those systems. Indeed, we have yet to establish a rich understanding of the processes of professional nursing practice.

On the other hand, technology has been a major driver in the development of information systems, resulting in systems that leverage available technology and technological advances. However, these systems are not reflective of the workflow and decision-making processes of healthcare professionals. Similarly, the concept of human factors has not been well defined or incorporated into information system design. Today's technology-driven information systems foster patterns of adoption that are the result of the technological characteristics of the system, rather than the use of the system to appropriately support workflow and decision-making processes. Widespread adoption of numerous technologies into day-to-day life has clearly occurred; however, in health care, we are only beginning to use the potential of information systems. Still, the design of information systems today is not based on process understanding; consequently, system utilization has been limited.

In addition to the insight that system requirements have not been grounded in process understanding, further analysis has uncovered another inadequacy of the original framework related to knowledge-driven systems. Blum (1986) put forth the definitions of data, information, and knowledge that have since guided nursing informatics:

- *Data*—Discrete entities that are described objectively without interpretation.
- *Information*—Data that are interpreted, organized, or structured.
- *Knowledge*—Information that has been synthesized so that interrelationships are identified and formalized.

(Because Blum was the primary referent in the early scholarship of nursing informatics, we have limited our source to Blum. We acknowledge that much scholarship has been done on expanding understanding of the concepts of data, information, and knowledge since Blum's work.)

The original framework for this monograph, as well as the thinking in the early 1990s, failed to adequately take into account the concept of knowledge. A key insight in formulating a vision and recommendations for the future is the fundamental role of knowledge generation, dissemination, and validation in nursing practice and within the information systems that support this practice.

Information, viewed as organized data, guides the clinician and supports critical thinking and decision-making. To do this effectively within the complex, adaptive healthcare system, information must be given context, and be timely, relevant, complete, actionable, and amenable to manipulation. In every clinical encounter the clinician integrates all available external information with the clinician's existing internal knowledge base.

Argyris (1993) describes a ladder of inference, where an individual examines directly observable data and incorporates culturally shared meaning to make judgments and draw inferences, thus building beliefs and assumptions. A reflexive loop involuntarily affects the process by allowing our beliefs to directly influence the selection process by which we receive new observable data. According to Wheatley (1994, p. 36), "Self-organizing systems have the capacity for continuous change because they have access to the intelligence that exists everywhere within them." Thus, clinical information systems of the future must support the user by providing data at the point of decision-making that are structured to facilitate the extraction of critical knowledge; indiscriminant and irrelevant data may actually impair decision making. "Professional knowledge is not facts or information... it is the application of knowledge through the use of critical thinking skills" (Eisenhauer 1998, p. 52).

As our knowledge has expanded to incorporate the influential forces, interactions, current environment, and future we envision, the framework has changed. The new framework, derived from the original, integrates the concepts of knowledge-driven systems, the iterative nature of data, information, and knowledge, and the use of knowledge in nursing practice to validate existing knowledge and generate new knowledge. A key point that emerges from this work is that validating, synthesizing, and generating knowledge is the raison d'être for adopting information systems into nursing practice environments.

Chapter 1 identified the fourth phase of CIS development. This phase focuses on flow-driven systems that bring together knowledge, decision-making enhancements, and improvements in workflow support that can lead to effective and efficient health care. Healthcare practitioners now recognize that useful information systems foster collaboration and cooperation by bringing together and integrating all clinical information.

Note how Figure 5-1 depicts the position of clinical knowledge and its relationship to the clinical information system. This evolution in thinking significantly influences the identification of recommendations for the next steps in the design, development, implementation, and evaluation of clinical information systems for professional nursing practice.

Next Steps

The authors of this monograph acknowledge that many of the key specifications and recommendations to achieve a system reflective of this vision and new framework have been well described (IOM 1991, 1997, 2000, 2001; Raymond and Dold 2002; see also Appendix A). Rather than repeating that which has been documented

Figure 5-1. Organizing Framework for Clinical Information Systems: Clinical Knowledge as Critical Factor

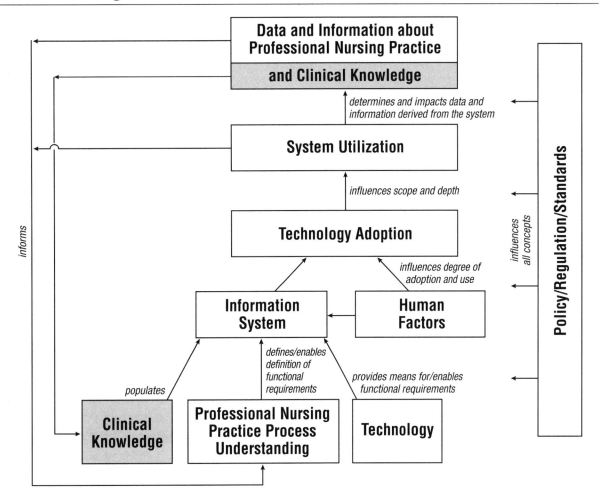

elsewhere, the following section focuses on leadership and disruptive innovation as key strategies to achieve these previously cited recommendations as well as those recommended in this document.

Much has been written in the past 10 years about leadership and change management—the inevitability of change and the critical role of leaders in assuring that organizations not only tolerate, but also prosper in the face of change. This is familiar content, yet there remains a real void in the type of leadership and the type of change necessary to achieve the described vision.

In Chapter 4, we referenced the Christensen, Bohmer and Kenagy work (2000), in which they discuss the need for disruptive innovation, defined as "...disruptive technologies and business models that may threaten the status quo but will ultimately raise the quality of care for everyone" (p. 104). These authors state that the types and characteristics of change that the culture of health care welcomes are not those that will result in achieving the vision we have identified. Rather, the welcomed changes are those that will reinforce the political, organizational, and financial framework in which care is currently provided. A key to understanding the premise of disruptive innovation is realizing where such innovation is targeted. "Many of the most powerful innovations that disrupted other industries did so by enabling a larger population of less-skilled people to do in a more convenient, less expensive setting things that historically could be performed only by expensive specialists in centralized, inconvenient locations" (Christensen, Bohmer, and Kenagy 2000, p. 105). The history of the development of personal computing is a classic example of such innovation. The tasks that in the 1960s required finding and accessing a mainframe computer and its associated skilled personnel can now be performed by more than 50% of our population at home in their pajamas.

We must innovate and change the use of technology in health care in comparable ways. Nursing leaders must foster the use of technology to expand, not control, the contributions of patients and nonphysician providers to the process of care. "Rather than ask complex, high-cost institutions and expensive, specialized professionals to move down-market, we need to look at the problem in a very different way. We need innovation that enables procedures to be done in less expensive, more convenient settings" (Christensen, Bohmer, and Kenagy 2000, pp. 105–106).

Functioning in a leadership role in today's highly complex healthcare environment requires visionary leaders. "Instead of working to preserve the existing system, healthcare regulators need to ask how they can enable disruptive innovations to emerge" (Christensen, Bohmer, and Kenagy 2000, p. 112). Leadership in healthcare organizations of the twenty-first century demands competent nurses with different skill sets than in the past. These leaders must understand systems as well as the distinctions between replicating existing processes in automated systems versus using systems as a tool to improve processes. Planning for continuous improvement and process redesign of quality, service and cost-effectiveness are critical competencies of successful twenty-first century healthcare leaders.

Nursing is perhaps the best-positioned discipline in the healthcare system to lead this type of disruptive innovation and change. We have a long history of demonstrating the capacity to not only adapt to, but also to lead, the instances of disruptive innovation in health care. Our nurse practitioner colleagues have both anecdotally and statistically demonstrated the positive impact of such innovation. As another example, nurses have helped diabetic patients demonstrate the potential for such change through the patients' ability to use technology in the home setting.

To accelerate the adoption of such innovative change, different leadership strategies are needed. Senge and colleagues (1994), in their work on learning organizations, explore five disciplines that are critical to organizational learning—learning that is consistent with an environment in which disruptive innovation is not only tolerated but also demanded (p. 307). One of the five disciplines is personal mastery (Senge et al. 1994, p. 6). Personal mastery is defined as "learning to expand our personal capacity to create results we most desire, and creating an organizational environment which encourages all its members to develop themselves toward the goals and purposes they choose." Fundamental to the discipline of personal mastery is the recognition that no individual can increase another's personal mastery, but must manage his or her own. Key steps in personal mastery include defining personal vision, acknowledging current reality, and taking steps to choose results and actions that move toward closer alignment of vision and current reality. Personal mastery represents a complex set of thoughts and perspectives, although in many ways it seems quite simple. Only by honestly facing one's own personal and professional vision and current reality can a leader have a basis for recognizing and choosing otherwise unavailable results and actions: unavailable, because they would be unrecognizable.

Unlike the current environment in which we have made limited progress in achieving our vision for clinical information systems, we believe that those leaders and organizations who can truly acknowledge their vision (as the IOM has) and objectively and honestly define the current reality, will identify the opportunities for disruptive, creative, and truly exciting innovation in the use of technology. This will then become the means for achieving their vision.

Next Steps: Strategies

In light of these insights regarding leadership and disruptive innovation, critical strategies for implementing these recommendations include the following.

Vision-driven Leadership

- Move beyond a reworking and reorganizing of traditional ideas and concepts that have not worked. Embrace new ideas that support the vision. Forget consensus—lead!
- Demand information systems that incorporate evidence-based knowledge into workflow at all points of care delivery.
- Demonstrate respect for nurses' critical thinking and subsequent reflective documentation by creating a feedback mechanism that facilitates system modifications.
- Recognize the expanding role of the informatics nurse specialist as a resource with the knowledge and skills necessary to identify and implement innovative solutions.

Identification of Concrete Disruptive Innovations

- Consider creative solutions and embrace change. Advocate rebellion against the status quo in nursing practice processes and clinical information systems.
- Center innovations around the relationship of the clinician and the patient and consider the need for embracing a new culture.
- Insist that all workflow innovations, including CIS, provide benefits to users that support the vision and reinforce new behaviors.

Research and Demonstration Projects

- Use prototyping methodology to explore specific ways to realize innovations.
- Pilot test technology-based innovations and new workflow processes. Do not be afraid to try, evaluate, and revise.
- Fund research that captures the distinctive thinking, practices, and outcomes of successful and unsuccessful disruptive change efforts.
- Demonstrate to nurses and other clinicians that adding to our body of knowledge is a significant payoff from documentation.

Next Steps: Actions

This section presents recommended actions to achieve this vision. These recommendations are organized in the following categories:

- Implementing our knowledge and learnings
- Learning new skills and approaches
- Redesigning aspects of our systems

Implementing Our Knowledge and Learnings

As discussed in Chapter 4, there is a pattern in the development and implementation of clinical information systems of *not* leveraging our knowledge and learnings. Although the discipline of healthcare informatics is relatively young, a significant body of knowledge and experience exists that, if utilized, would impact how systems are developed and implemented. When considering recommendations for this area, three key actions are available that, if consistently adopted, would result in the integration of past experience and knowledge into current efforts.

- First, in all instances, all phases of the software development lifecycle must be executed to include a systematic review of previous requirements, design, and use experience in the functional area the system is to address. For example, a software project to design the functionality to support care planning would include a systematic review of all experience and research in the area of design of care planning software. And, the findings from the review would be conscientiously incorporated in the next design of the software.
- Second, a similar pattern of systematic review must be executed as part of the implementation process for other clinical software.
- And third, and perhaps in some ways most fundamental, healthcare informatics education must explicitly incorporate the available content from experience and research and identify the associated implications. The best practices for system development and implementation can then be identified, researched, and translated into competencies.

It is noteworthy that the authors are recommending that the feedback loop of the organizing framework should be described in terms of utilization, dissemination, and validation of clinical knowledge be applied to clinical systems knowledge.

Learning New Skills and Approaches

As discussed throughout this monograph, business modeling, complex project management, team leadership and participation, communication, and change management are critical skills in the development and implementation of clinical information systems. Significant progress has been made in recognizing these skills as basic nursing informatics competencies (ANA 2001). However, nursing education and practice have not recognized business and process modeling as core competencies necessary to the design and implementation of information systems that truly support and improve clinical processes. In addition to the integration of existing experiential and research knowledge described, the skills that appear to be most critical to achieving the vision are the use of formal modeling techniques in the development of clinical systems. New skills and approaches must consider and incorporate the potential and value of object-oriented modeling, which has been demonstrated in isolated instances of terminology and process redesign work.

Redesigning Aspects of Our Systems

The recommended actions related to implementation of knowledge and learning, and the adoption of new skills and approaches, provide the context for the recommended actions to support redesign of aspects of our systems. The following recommendations related to clinical information system design call for commitment by the individual, organization, and profession to:

- Support the development and adoption of healthcare vocabulary and data exchange standards.
- Demand that evidence-based structured databases be included in any clinical information system
- Demand that information systems developers ground their work on professional nursing practice understanding represented in formal models.
- Use research-based evidence of nurses' information seeking behaviors in the clinical information design.
- Expect that business process modeling techniques be adopted for information system design.
- Design systems based on the fundamental understanding of the distinctions between process automation, process improvement, and process reengineering.

Conclusions

In the concluding chapter of *Next-Generation Nursing Information Systems: Essential Characteristics for Professional Practice* (1993), the authors asserted that a comprehensive solution to clinical nursing's information management needs had not yet been identified, developed, and implemented. They anticipated that the *Next-Generation* document's contribution would be in identifying the necessary context for successful implementation and the characteristics and features of the next generation of nursing information systems. The authors also advocated for leadership and collaboration to ensure that (p. 51):

- "nursing knowledge feeds nursing information systems and vice versa;
- NISs [nursing information systems] meet the needs of nurse users;
- nursing speaks with a unified voice to system developers; and,
- nursing information will fit within the context of a total integrated patient record system."

Now, 10 years later, nurses still await the reality of a solution to meet their information management needs, but progress is being made. The authors of this monograph propose a framework for representing the concepts and relationships for successful clinical information system implementations that support practice. This organizing framework for clinical information systems (diagrammed in Figure 5-1 on page 51) depicts the integral components and feedback loops for:

- clinical knowledge,
- professional nursing practice process understanding,
- technology,
- human factors, and
- the information system.

The framework also identifies the associated relationships of:

- technology adoption,
- system utilization,
- policy, regulation, and standards, and
- data and information about professional nursing practice and clinical knowledge.

This framework can help guide the design, development, implementation, and evaluation of information systems that truly support the workflow and knowledge generation required for integration in nursing practice.

Certainly the health care environment is very different now in 2003, and the need for visionary leaders is thus even more critical. These leaders—by using the framework described and applying disruptive innovation techniques—can make the vision of the future a reality. That reality will be the realization of the two complimentary goals for all operational clinical information systems: to support and enable change, and to serve as transforming and powerful tools. The end result: nurses in all domains of professional practice will have the data, information, and knowledge resources needed to inform their work to provide quality healthcare.

References

ANA (American Nurses Association). 2001. *The Scope and Standards of Informatics Nursing Practice.* Washington, DC: American Nurses Publishing.

Argyris, C. 1993. In Kim DH. Transformational leadership: The leader with the "beginner's mind." *Healthcare Forum Journal* 36(4): 32–37.

Blum, B. I. 1986. *Clinical Information Systems.* New York: Springer-Verlag.

Christensen, C. M., R. Bohmer, and J. Kenagy. 2000. Will disruptive innovations cure health care? *Harvard Business Review* September–October: 102–110.

IOM (Institute of Medicine). 1991. *The Computer-based Patient Record: An Essential Technology for Change.* (Dick, R.S., and E. B. Steen). Washington, DC: Institute of Medicine.

———. 1997. *The Computer-based Patient Record—An Essential Technology for Health Care, rev. ed.* (Dick, R.S., E. B. Steen, and D. E. Detmer, eds.). Washington, DC: National Academy Press.

———. 2000. *To Err Is Human.* Committee on Quality of Health Care in America. Washington, DC: National Academy Press.

———. 2001. *Crossing the Quality Chasm.* Washington, DC: National Academy Press.

Eisenhauer, L. 1998. The reconstruction of professional knowledge. *Journal of Nursing Education* 37(2): 51–52.

Raymond, B., and C. Dold. 2002. *Clinical Information Systems: Achieving the Vision.* Oakland, CA: Kaiser Permanente Institute for Health Policy.

Senge, P. M., A. Kleiner, C. Roberts, R. B. Ross, and B. J. Smith. 1994. *The Fifth Discipline Handbook.* New York: Doubleday.

Wheatley, M. 1994. *Leadership and the New Science: Learning About Organizations From an Orderly Universe.* San Francisco: Berrett-Koehler.

Zielstorff, R., C. Hudgings, and S. Grobe. 1993. *Next-Generation Nursing Information Systems: Essential Characteristics for Professional Practice.* Washington, DC: American Nurses Publishing.

Next-Generation Assumptions & Criteria

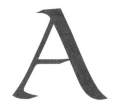

(From Zielstorff, R., C. Hudgings, and S. Grobe. 1993. *Next-Generation Nursing Information Systems: Essential Characteristics for Professional Practice*. Washington, DC: American Nurses Publishing.)

ASSUMPTIONS

		Criteria met today	Criteria still relevant today
1	The NIS exists within the context of a total integrated patient-record system. (p. 5)	Yes	Yes
2	Health care is an information-intensive industry. (p. 5)	Yes	Yes
3	Information is a critical resource in the health care environment. (p. 6)	Yes	Yes
4	Nursing practice is essentially an information-processing activity. (p. 6)	Yes	Yes
5	Systems integration is an essential part of a successful NIS. (p. 6)	Yes	Yes
6	Patient-specific data are the focal point of a totally integrated patient-record system. (p. 6)	Yes	Yes
7	Atomic-level data, captured in the NIS, will be used for many purposes. (p. 7)	No	Yes
8	Data and data elements required for a nursing information system will evolve. (p. 8)	Yes	Yes
9	Information technologies allow us not merely to replicate a manual system, but to process data differently. (p. 8)	No	Yes
10	For the foreseeable future, nursing will continue to have multiple theoretical frameworks, lexicons, data dictionaries, and models. (p. 8)	Yes	Yes
11	Technologies will be developed to bridge multiple lexicons. (p. 9)	Some progress	Yes
12	Clinical nursing will continue to have a large textual component. (p. 9)	Yes	Yes
13	To ensure high-quality practice, nurses need access to sources of data that are beyond institutional, patient-specific data. (p. 9)	No	Yes
14	There will always be a need for human interpretation of computer-processed data. (p. 9)	Yes	Yes
15	Users of an integrated patient-centered system will be professionally diverse. (p. 10)	Yes	Yes
16	Technology will continue to evolve in ways that make information systems for professionals more useful. (p. 10)	Yes	Yes
17	Education will equip nurses to be more sophisticated in using computer technology to support delivery of care and clinical decision making. (p. 11)	No	Yes

FUNCTIONAL REQUIREMENTS: GOALS	Criteria met	Criteria relevant
18 The system must promote efficiency and productivity. (p. 13)	Some progress	Yes
19 The system must promote effectiveness of care by assisting clinicians to make the best possible decisions for their clients. (p. 13)	Some progress	Yes

FUNCTIONAL REQUIREMENTS: SYSTEM CHARACTERISTICS

	Criteria met	Criteria relevant
20 Flexibility: The system must be able to be configured at the implementation site with respect to conceptual framework or nursing model, structured vocabulary, displays and reports, and decision rules. (p. 14)	Some progress	Yes
21 Flexibility: The system must be able to be upgraded as new technological developments become available. To every extent possible, upgrades to the system should enable transferability of existing data to the new system. (p. 14)	Yes	Yes
22 Flexibility: The system must be able to respond to changing requirements in methods of delivering care, and in methods of reporting to external agencies. (p. 14)	Yes	Yes
23 Connectivity: The system should be able to communicate with other information systems within the agency to reduce redundant data entry and avoid duplicate databases. (p. 14)	Some progress	Yes
24 Connectivity: The system should be able to support standard and evolving communication protocols to enable data sharing among otherwise disparate systems. (p. 14)	Yes	Yes
25 Connectivity: The system should be able to provide communication links to external systems such as bibliographic retrieval systems, data banks, and other knowledge resources. (p. 14)	Yes	Yes
26 Connectivity: The system should be able to acquire data from other systems, and be able to contribute data to other systems and agencies (to support a longitudinal patient record, for example, or to contribute data to a national database for inquiry or research). (p. 14)	Yes	Yes
27 Performance: The system should demonstrate satisfactory performance (according to bench-mark criteria) at peak calculated work-load times. (p. 14)	Yes	Yes
28 Performance: The system should provide continuous service (no downtime), as when the system is implemented with "non-stop technology" or with redundant back-up systems. (p. 14)	Yes	Yes
29 Security and confidentiality: Integrity of all data should be assured, so that data are captured, transmitted, stored, and displayed without error. Mechanisms for assuring data integrity would be described and demonstrable. (p. 14)	Yes	Yes
30 Security and confidentiality: Data should be protected from unauthorized access by means of security codes and or other unique user identifiers. (p. 14)	Yes	Yes
31 Security and confidentiality: Audit trails should be kept of all transactions that alter data within the patient's record, including date, time, and identity of person carrying out the action. Entries subsequently marked as erroneous should be kept — not deleted — and flagged as erroneous, with the usual audit notations. (p. 14)	Yes	Yes
32 Security and confidentiality: Confidentiality of patient and provider data should be protected. There are many ways to do this. Some are as simple as not leaving a patient's data displayed on the screen for more than a certain number of seconds, unless there is verification that someone is still using it. Other methods involve more complex algorithms that either strip or encrypt unique patient and provider identifiers before sending the patient's record to a larger database for research or inquiry. (p. 15)	Yes	Yes

	Criteria met	Criteria relevant

33 Human factors: The system must be able to accommodate a variety of data capture methods, each best suited to the circumstance and the type of data being captured. In general, the principle that data should be captured as close to the time and source of creation as possible should be followed. For some types of data, bar code readers will be most efficient; for others, touch screens, light pens, pen pads, mouse, or voice recognition will be more appropriate. Miniature hand-held terminals will be most appropriate for some tasks and settings, while lap-top portable terminals may be best for others, such as home visits. (p. 15) — *Some progress* / *Yes*

34 Human factors: Data capture methods must be no more time-consuming than manual methods for entering comparable data. To the extent possible, the automated system should be less time-consuming to use than the comparable manual system. (p. 15) — *No* / *Yes*

35 Human factors: The theoretical framework for the nursing process and the vocabulary to be used should be configurable at the site. Preferably, these will be determined by local professional consensus. The site should not be forced to use a particular framework simply because the system purchased is designed to work only with that framework. (p. 15) — *Some progress* / *Yes*

36 Human factors: The system's user-interface design should follow established principles of user/machine dialogue. Consumers may have difficulty evaluating this system characteristic. Generally, some important principles have been incorporated if the dialogue sequence seems to make sense intuitively, without a lot of explanation of what to do next; if relevant information is displayed with enough detail to inform without overwhelming at first glance; and if help and error messages are presented in clear, helpful, "non-jargon" phrases. (p. 15) — *Some progress* / *Yes*

37 Human factors: Connections to other systems — whether internal or external to the agency — should appear "seamless" to the user. Incorporating all the access codes and log-on scripts within a master menu on the main system is desirable. The user would then simply choose an application and be logged on to the appropriate system. (p. 15) — *No* / *Yes*

USABILITY PRINCIPLES FOR USER INTERFACES

38 Simple and natural dialogue. Dialogues should not contain information that is irrelevant or rarely needed. Every extra unit of information in a dialogue competes with the relevant units of information and diminishes their relative visibility. All information should appear in a natural and logical order. (p. 16) — *Yes* / *Yes*

39 Speak the users' language. The dialogue should be expressed clearly in words, phrases, and concepts familiar to the user, rather than in system-oriented terms. (p. 16) — *Yes* / *Yes*

40 Minimize the users' memory load. The user should not have to remember information from one part of the dialogue to another. Instructions for use of the system should be visible or easily retrievable whenever appropriate. (p. 16) — *Yes* / *Yes*

41 Consistency. Users should not have to wonder whether words, situations, and actions mean the same thing. (p. 16) — *Yes* / *Yes*

42 Provide feedback. The system should always keeps users informed about what is going on through appropriate feedback within reasonable time. (p. 16) — *Yes* / *Yes*

43 Provide clearly marked exits. Users often choose system functions by mistake and will need a clearly marked "emergency exit" to leave the unwanted state without having to go through an extended dialogue. (p. 16) — *Yes* / *Yes*

44 Provide shortcuts. Clever shortcuts — unseen by the novice user — may often speed up the interaction for the expert user such that the system caters to both inexperienced and experienced users. (p. 16) — *Yes* / *Yes*

45 Good error messages. Error message should be expressed in plain language (no codes), precisely indicate the problem, and constructively suggest a solution. (p. 16) — *Yes* / *Yes*

46 Prevent errors. Even better than good error messages is a careful design that prevents a problem from occurring in the first place. (p. 16) — *Yes* / *Yes*

DESIGN CONSIDERATIONS: PATIENT-SPECIFIC DATA	*Criteria met*	*Criteria relevant*
47 Acquiring: The system must be able to capture all patient data the nurse needs for patient care. (p. 20)	No	Yes
48 Acquiring: Patient data capture should be structured, to the greatest degree possible, with accepted vocabularies, dictionaries, and lexicons. (p. 20)	No	Yes
49 Acquiring: The system must be able to capture all data generated by the nurse in the course of patient care, as close to the time and place of creation as possible, and in the most efficient manner possible. (p. 20)	No	Yes
50 Acquiring: Patient data should be captured at their source. (p. 20)	No	Yes
51 Storing: Patient-specific data should be stored independently of the programs that capture the data. (p. 21)	Yes	Yes
52 Storing: Data elements should be structured so they can server multiple users and multiple purposes. (p. 21)	Yes	Yes
53 Storing: Unlimited keys for indexing the data should be allowed. (p. 21)	Yes	Yes
54 Transforming: The system should have the capability of transforming data to information, and information to knowledge. (p. 21)	No	Yes
55 Transforming: The system should be capable of mapping to and from various constructs and vocabularies. (p. 21)	Some progress	Yes
56 Presenting: The system should accommodate the level of expertise of the practitioner. (p. 22)	No	Yes
57 Presenting: Data, information, and knowledge should be presented in the format most suitable to assist decision-making. (p. 22)	No	Yes
58 Presenting: The system should be able to tailor "views" of the data to various disciplines, and should support ad hoc queries from end users. (p. 22)	Yes	Yes
59 Presenting: The system should be able to transform data according to practice models in use. (p. 22)	No	Yes
60 Presenting: Data, information, and knowledge presented to middle- or upper-level management should be derived from atomic-level data. (p. 23)	Some progress	Yes
DESIGN CONSIDERATIONS: AGENCY-SPECIFIC DATA		
61 Acquiring: General considerations; the same design considerations apply as were described for patient-specific data. (p. 23)	No	Yes
62 Acquiring: The system should accommodate entry of all of the agency's policy and procedure manuals. (p. 23)	No	Yes
63 Acquiring: The information system should accommodate standardized care plans and other structured models (such as critical pathways) appropriate to the agency. (p. 23)	Some progress	Yes
64 Acquiring: The system should accommodate information on the agency's departments, personnel, inventories, and services as needed for patient care. (p. 23)	No	Yes
65 Storing: Text-based data should be structured and stored with appropriate technology to facilitate comprehension and retrievability. (p. 24)	No	Yes
66 Storing: Data should be structured to enhance single-entry, multiple use. (p. 24)	Yes	Yes
67 Transforming: The system should be able to apply policies, standards, protocols, and guidelines to patient-specific data, to enhance clinical decision making and facilitate patient care. (p. 24)	No	Yes
68 Presenting: The system should present data rapidly, in the form most suitable for assistance in patient care and clinical decision making. (p. 24)	Some progress	Yes

		Criteria met	*Criteria relevant*
69	Presenting: Regardless of where agency-specific data are housed, they should be available through NIS. (p. 25)	Some progress	Yes
70	Presenting: The system should be able to tailor views of the data to various users and purposes, and should support ad hoc queries from end users. (p. 25)	No	Yes
71	Presenting: The system should be able to control access to data, based on "need to know." (p. 25)	Yes	Yes

DESIGN CONSIDERATIONS: DOMAIN-SPECIFIC INFORMATION AND KNOWLEDGE

72	Acquiring: The NIS should be capable of storing permanently whatever practice-related data of the agency has the potential of becoming domain-specific information. (p. 25)	No	Yes
73	Acquiring: The NIS should be able to incorporate domain-specific rules of practice into the logic of the patient information system to provide real-time clinical decision assistance. (p. 25)	No	Yes
74	Acquiring: The information system should be able to access bibliographic retrieval resources directly at the locus of care. (p. 26)	Yes	Yes
75	Acquiring: The system should connect to other available external sources of knowledge. (p. 26)	Yes	Yes
76	Storing: The system should store the agency's practice-related data as a structured database, capable of being manipulated, analyzed, and queried. (p. 26)	No	Yes
77	Storing: The domain-specific knowledge stored at the agency should be catalogued and well indexed, with established mechanisms of review and regular updating by qualified experts. (p. 27)	No	Yes
78	Transforming: The NIS should be able to apply systems that incorporate domain-specific knowledge directly to patient-specific data, or be able to export patient-specific data in a variety of standard formats. (p. 27)	No	Yes
79	Transforming: A variety decision-assistance tools that transform data into information, information into knowledge, and knowledge into new knowledge and decisions should be made available to the nurse at the locus of care. (p. 27)	No	Yes
80	Presenting: There should be a variety of ways to deliver domain-specific information and knowledge, depending on the source and the purpose. (p. 27)	No	Yes
81	Presenting: Domain-specific information and knowledge should be presented in the form most suitable to assist assimilation and decision assistance. (p. 27)	No	Yes

CONDITIONS BASIC TO SUCCESS

82	Evolution and Maturation of Nursing's Knowledge Base (p. 35)	Some progress	Yes
83	An Environmental Context of Administrative Support (p. 36)	Some progress	Yes
84	Standards for Clinical Data and Data Communication (p. 37)	Some progress	Yes
85	Cadre of Knowledgeable Nurses (p. 41)	Some progress	Yes
86	Collaboration Between Nurses and System Developers (p. 42)	Some progress	Yes

HIMSS Annual Leadership Surveys 1990–2002

B

	1990	1991	1992
Most important IT priority next 1–2 yrs.	Integrating existing systems	Integrating existing systems	Integrating existing systems
Most significant force driving computerization/ Top business issue	Improving the quality of patient care	Optimize overall efficiency of hospital	Containing healthcare costs
Desired advance in computer technology/ Most rapid growth	Systems integration	Friendlier user interface	Integrated voice/data technology
Most frustrating IT problem/ Significant barrier			
Greatest investment/Most important IT project	Patient care/bedside systems	Patient care/bedside systems	Patient care/bedside systems
Important technology of the future	"Medical 'credit card' (smart card) will happen by the year 2000"	Open systems	Optical scanning
Investment in clinical information/Point of care systems		15% (primarily in critical care units)	17% (primarily in critical care units)
Progress toward implementing a CPR			"It's a promising concept but practical application still 5–10 yrs away"
Information technology terms of the year	"Medical" 'credit card' (smart card), integration, HL7, Medix, interface"	"DOS, Unix, mainframe, minicomputer, pc, workstation"	"Voice processing, cabling/wiring technology, PC LANs, PACS"

1993	1994	1995
Integrating existing systems	Integrating systems across facilities	Integrating systems across facilities Upgrade IT infrastructure
Government and payer pressure to control costs	Movement to managed care	Movement to managed care
"User input/output devices (e.g. voice, pen)"	Clinical data repository	Clinical data repository
	Lack of strategic IT plan	Lack of strategic IT plan
	Integrating systems across separate facilities	
Wireless LAN	Pen-based systems	Multimedia
26% (primarily in critical care units)	33% (primarily in critical care units)	37% (primarily in critical care units)
It will be a reality within the next 5 years	"Still evaluating options, No decisions have been made"	"Still evaluating options, No decisions have been made"
"Fiber optics, ISDN, Wireless LAN, 4th generation PBX, video conferencing, EDI, HL7, Microsoft NT"	"Internet, client/server, passwords, point of care, clinical data repositories, case management, outcomes analysis tools, Ethernet"	"Telemedicine, multimedia, point of care, Ethernet, ATM, Token Ring, Wireless LAN"

	1996	1997	1998
Most important IT priority next 1–2 yrs.	Upgrade IT infrastructure	Upgrade IT infrastructure	Recruit and retain high-quality IT staff
Most significant force driving computerization/ Top business issue	Need to control costs due to pressure from managed care	Drive to achieve competitive advantage in the market	Deriving more value from existing data
Desired advance in computer technology/ Most rapid growth	Clinical data repository	Clinical data repository	
Most frustrating IT problem - Significant barrier	Lack of strategic IT plan	Lack of strategic IT plan	Lack of adequate financial support for IT
Greatest investment/Most important IT project	Upgrade IT infrastructure	Upgrade IT infrastructure	
Important technology of the future	Smart cards	Web-enabled applications	Voice recognition
Investment in clinical information/Point of care systems			
Progress toward implementing a CPR	Have a strategic plan but haven't made any investments	Have invested substantially in equipment/software	Planning or installing a CPR (44%)
Information technology terms of the year	"Telemedicine, CHIN, Worldwide Web, Ethernet, Token Ring, Wireless LAN, ATM, FDDI, smart card, clinical data repository"	"Intranet, HTML, HL7, DICOM, multimedia, distance education, object-oriented technology, wireless information appliances"	"Firewall, encryption, Y2K, telecommunications, token based authentication, plug and play, digital signatures, handheld PDA"

1999	2000	2001	2002
Implement a Y2K conversion	Deployment of Internet technology/HIPAA compliance	Upgrade security/HIPAA compliance	Upgrade security/HIPAA compliance
	HIPAA compliance	HIPAA compliance	HIPAA compliance
	Clinical information systems	Clinical information systems	Clinical information systems
Difficulty recruiting and retaining high-quality IT staff	Difficulty in providing IT quantifiable benefits/return on investment	Lack of adequate financial support for IT	Lack of adequate financial support for IT
	Clinical information systems	Clinical information systems	Clinical information systems
Wireless information appliances	E-business	Wireless information appliances	Wireless information appliances
Planning or installing a CPR (68%)	Planning or installing a CPR (64%)	Planning or installing a CPR (66%)	Planning or installing CPR (68%)
"e-business, voice recognition, data mining, handheld PDA, smartcard, HIPAA, telehealth"	"E-health, MPI, Enterprise Resource Planning (ERP) systems, client-server, Thin clients, XML, Extranet, Web-enabled business transactions, ASP"	"Digital certificates, PKI, biometrics, wireless, data warehouse, extranet, handheld PDAs, client-server, web-enabled transactions, voice recognition, XML, ASP"	"Enterprise resource planning (ERP), Internet technology, security tools, firewall, off-site storage, PKI, handheld devices, voice recognition, ASP, outsourcing"

Twenty Years of History:
Nursing Informatics at SCAMC/AMIA

C

History of Nursing at SCAMC/AMIA

- 1981: First Nursing Track at SCAMC (Society for Computer Applications in Medical Care)
- 1981–1990: NI SIG at SCAMC
- 1990: SIG moves to AMIA
- 1994: Nurse chairs Program Committee
- 1998: Nurse elected President
- 2001: Nurse is President; Nurse chairs Program Committee

Nursing Administration

- 1973: First Invitational Conference of Management Information Systems for Public Health/Community Health (NLN)
- 1974–1975: Follow-up workshops
- 1977: First Research Conference on Nursing Information Systems
- 1981–2000: Over 250 published journal articles related to using computers to address administrative concerns

Nursing Practice

- 1981–1982: First national and international conferences
- 1984: First journal
- 1986: Nursing Minimum Data Set (NMDS) Conference in Milwaukee
- 1988: NIH Priority Expert Panel
- 1991: ICN International Classification of Nursing Practice
- 1992: ANA identifies Nursing Informatics specialty and standards
- 1993: Nursing Languages included in NLM-Unified Medical Language System (UMLS)
- 1996: ANA Nursing Information and Data Set Evaluation Center (NIDSEC)
- 1999–2002: Nursing Vocabulary Summit Conferences

Nursing Education
- 1977: First course in Informatics
- 1984: First textbook
- 1987: Guidelines in Computer Education
- 1988: IMIA Nursing Informatics Competencies
- 1988–1991 (to 2001): Initial development of graduate degrees
- 1998: Information technology competencies for accreditation

By the Decades: Changes of Focus
A proposed clinical nursing practice/informatics focus by decade is as follows (Romano, 2001):
- 1980: Automation
- 1990: Info-mation
- 2000: Communication and Integration
- 2010: Knowledge Creation

Evolution of Informatics
These informatics themes have evolved over the past years, moving from:
- Data cemetery to knowledge repository
- Data entry to data extraction
- Documentation to decision support
- Text to vocabularies/taxonomies
- Information silos to integrated networks
- Technology for convenience to safety and outcomes
- Disciplinary to interdisciplinary
- Provider resource to consumer resource

Note: This table is constructed from presentations at the AMIA 2001 Panel, "20 Years of Nursing at SCAMC/AMIA." Participants: J. Ozbolt, P. Button, V. Saba, K. McCormick, C. Delaney, C. Romano, J. Ronald, and P. Brennan.

Index

Computerized physician order entry (CPOE), 32, 35
    See also Order processing
Confidentiality. *See* Data security
Connectivity, 15, 20, 36
    Next Generation criteria, 18, 62, 65
Coordinated care, 36
    See also Patient care
Cost controls, 13, 34
    priority of, 9, 10, 14, 31, 32, 54, 68, 69, 70
Council on Computer Applications in Nursing. *See under* American Nurses Association
Crossing the Quality Chasm (IOM 2001), 31, 32, 43, 44, 46

D

Data analysis, 50
    patient outcomes, 10, 11, 23, 32, 33, 35
    workflow, 9, 11, 36
Data capture, 20, 21, 34
    impediments to, 38
    data entry formats, 17, 37
    historical emphasis on, 8–9
    Next Generation criteria, 63, 64, 65
    nursing and, 10, 30
    standards and, 14, 32
    See also Bar codes; Data Capture; Pen Pads; Touch Screens; Mouse; Voice recognition
Data communication
    electronic data interchange (EDI), 14, 16, 19, 32
    Next Generation criteria, 18, 62, 65
    priority of, 11, 15, 20, 30
Data encryption, 33
    Next Generation criteria, 18, 62
Data formats, 9, 15, 36, 57, 65
Data integration, 2–3, 50
    priority of, 19, 20, 30, 44
    See also Connectivity
Data integrity, 17, 20
    Next Generation criteria, 18, 62
Data quality, 19
Data re-use, 11, 35, 61, 64
Data security
    Next Generation criteria, 18, 62
    patient records, 15, 20, 43
    standards, 13, 32
    technologies, 33
Data sets, 11, 12, 51, 61
    NMDS, 8, 12, 23, 32, 73
    NMMDS, 36
Databases
    categories, 9, 11
    computer-based patient record, 15, 19–20
    Next Generation criteria, 18, 62, 65
    queries, 17

Decision support systems, 10–11, 35, 46, 51
    Next Generation criteria, 18, 62, 64, 65
    prerequisities for, 19, 30, 31
    priority of, 2, 9, 15, 16, 23, 52
Design considerations. *See* System design
Diagnosis-specific pathways, 30
Digital certificates, 33
    See also Data security
Digital imaging and communications in medicine (DICOM), 33, 36
    See also Image processing
Discovery methods, 15
Disruptive innovation, 47, 53–55, 58
Documentation of nursing practice, 12, 24, 55
    electronic storage of, 19, 30, 34, 43

E

Ease of use, 21, 37
    See also Human factors; Human-computer interaction; User interface
Education and skill development, 13, 16, 19, 56, 74
    nursing informatics, 8, 10, 31, 46, 49, 61
Efficiency. *See* Productivity
e-health, 34, 39
Electronic data interchange (EDI), 14, 16, 19, 32
Electronic signature, 14
Encryption. *See* Data encryption
Environment. *See* Healthcare industry characteristics
Ergonomics, 21, 32–33
    See also Human factors
Error messages, 63
    See also Usability
Error prevention. *See* Quality of care
Ethics and equity, 31, 33, 44
Evidence-based practice, 30, 35, 46, 55, 57
Expert systems, 23, 35
Extensible markup language (XML), 34

F

Feedback mechanisms, 49, 55, 56, 58

H

Handwriting recognition, 15, 23, 35
Hand-held terminals, 33, 38
    data capture via, 21, 37, 63
Harvard Business Review (on healthcare industry), 47
Health Insurance Portability and Accountability Act (HIPAA), 32, 71
Health Level 7 (HL7), 14, 33, 36
Healthcare Employer Data and Information Set (HEDIS), 14
    See also Data sets

Healthcare industry characteristics, 13, 25, 37–39
   nursing undervalued, 24
   priorities, 2–3, 14, 16, 31
   regulation, 32
   resistance to change, 47
   See also HIMSS Annual Leadership Survey
Healthcare Information and Management Systems Society (HIMSS), 7
   Annual Leadership Survey, 15, 23, 24, 35
      historical trends, 16, 20, 33–34, 67–71
      purpose, 13–14
Healthcare information systems
   historical background, 2–3, 4–5, 29–31
   models, 2–3
      data-driven, 2, 29, 45, 46
      workflow-driven, 2
      financial, 2
      order processing, 2
      See also Clinical information systems; Order processing; Workflow-driven systems
Help features, 21, 37, 63
   See also Usability
Human-computer interaction (HCI), 20, 33, 36, 37, 50
Human factors, 51
   in CIS organizing framework, 4, 5, 29, 44, 45, 58
   current status, 36–37
   definition of, 4, 20
   historical background, 20–22
   Next Generation criteria, 63
   See also Clinical information systems; Ergonomics; User interface
Human resource management, 9, 36, 64
Hypertext. *See* World Wide Web

I

Image processing, 15, 16, 50
   See also Digital imaging and communication in medicine
Independent nursing functions, 10
Inference engine. *See* Artificial intelligence; Knowledge-based systems
Informatics. *See* Nursing informatics
Information systems, 5, 29, 44, 58
   current status, 35–36
   definition of, 4
   historical background, 16–20
   See also Clinical information systems
Information technology, 14, 43–44
   See also Technology
Innovation and change, 31, 46, 47, 50, 52–55, 58
   See also Change management; Disruptive innovation
Institute of Medicine (IOM) research. *See The Computer-Based Patient Record*; *Crossing the Quality Chasm*; *To Err is Human*

Insurance. *See* Managed care
Integrated delivery networks (IDN), 36
Integrating the Healthcare Enterprise (IHE), 33
Interdependent nursing functions, 10
International Classification for Nursing Practice, 8, 32, 73
   See also Nursing language
International Council of Nurses (ICN), 8, 73
International Medical Informatics Association (IMIA), 22, 74
International Organization for Standardization (ISO), 33
Internet, 16, 33, 34, 37–38
Interventions, 10, 12
   recording, 9, 24, 30
Iterative design, 36, 37
   See also Software development

J

Joint Commission for Accreditation of Healthcare Organizations (JCAHO), 14, 32
Just-in-time information, 33

K

Knowledge. *See* Nursing knowledge
Knowledge-based systems, 15, 30, 35, 46, 51
   integration into clinical informations systems, 20, 34, 52

L

Laptop computers, 21, 37, 63
Leadership, 46, 56, 57
   and disruptive innovation, 47, 52–55
   See also Healthcare Information and Management Systems Society: Annual Leadership Survey
Learnings. *See* Nursing knowledge
Light pen, 21, 63, 69
Long Term Care Minimum Data Set, 32
   See also Data sets; Nursing languages

M

Managed care, 14, 30, 69
   and emphasis on cost control, 9, 31, 70
Messaging and alerts, 19, 30, 34, 35
Miniaturization, 21, 15, 63
Mobile computing, 34
   See also Laptop computers; Wireless devices
Model-based systems, 15
Modeling, , 45, 46
   business, 56–57
   object-oriented, 15–16
   Unified Modeling Language (UML), 34
   See also Prototyping

Models, 64
    best-practice, 30, 35
    nursing, 9, 18, 21, 30
    See also under Healthcare information systems
Mouse, 21, 33, 63
Multimedia, 15, 16, 69

N

National Center for Nursing Research (NCNR)
    Expert Panel on Nursing Informatics, 7, 8, 15, 21
    Research Priority Expert Panel on Nursing Informatics, 8–9
National Commission on Nursing Implementation Project (NCNIP), 1
National Committee for Quality Assurance (NCQA), 14, 32
National League for Nursing (NLN), 1, 8, 73
    Nursing Informatics Forum, 1
National Library of Medicine (NLM)
    Unified Medical Language System (UMLS), 8, 73
Natural language systems, 35
    See also Artificial intelligence; Knowledge-based systems
Networks, 15, 36, 43
    See also Connectivity
Next Generation Nursing Information Systems, iii, 5, 7, 57
    assumptions and criteria, 10, 11, 15, 16–19, 21, 22, 49, 50, 51, 61–66
    origins, 1–2
Nomenclature. *See* Nursing languages
Notebook computers. *See* Laptop computers
Nurse executivesand CISs, 36
Nursing
    clinical information systems and, 7–11, 24, 31, 65
    disruptive innovation and, 54–55
Nursing informatics, 45, 46, 55, 56
    history, 1–3, 73–74
    research, 7, 8, 13, 32–33, 51
Nursing Informatics: Enhancing Patient Care, 7, 23
Nursing Informatics Forum of NLN, 1
Nursing Informatics Working Group (NIWG) of AMIA, 1
Nursing Information and Data Set Evaluation Center (NIDSEC), 12, 73
Nursing information systems (NISs). *See* Clinical information systems
Nursing knowledge, 9, 58, 65
    dissemination, 50, 51–52
Nursing languages, 23, 43, 44, 73
    Next Generation criteria, 61, 63, 64
    requirements, 9, 12, 17, 18, 21, 25, 57
    standards, 14, 31, 32
Nursing Management Minimum Data Set (NMMDS), 36
    See also Data sets
Nursing Minimum Data Set (NMDS), 8, 12, 23, 32, 73
    See also Data sets; Nursing languages

Nursing models. *See under* Models
Nursing practice issues. *See* Professional nursing practice *entries*
Nursing process, 10, 21, 63
    CISs and, 16–18
Nursing taxonomy. *See* Nursing languages
Nursing Terminology Summit, 32, 33

O

Object-oriented design, 15, 34, 57
    See also Software development
Online systems, 16, 17, 30, 37
Open systems architecture, 16, 23, 68
Optical scanning, 68
Order processing, 10, 20, 29
    computerized physician order entry (CPOE), 32, 35
Organizational impacts of informatics (IMIA), 22, 74
Outcomes. *See* Patient outcomes

P

Pan American Health Organization (PAHO), 7, 23–24
Patient care, 32, 36, 46, 50
    CIS support of, 9, 20, 30, 31
    See also Coordinated care; Quality of care
Patient outcomes, 12, 19, 43
    analysis, 9, 10, 23, 32, 35
    See also under Data analysis
Patient records, 11, 16, 30, 31
    computer-based patient record (CPR), 13–15, 23, 25, 43, 68–71
    data security15, 20, 43
    Next Generation criteria, 61, 62, 64
    See also The Computer-Based Patient Record
Patient safety, 33, 35, 50
    priority of, 30, 31, 32, 44, 46
Pen pads, 21, 63
Performance
    system requirements, 17, 18, 19
    Next Generation criteria, 62
Personal computers, 16, 22, 37
Personal digital assistants (PDAs), 33
    See also Hand-held terminals
Personal mastery, 54
Planning, strategic. *See* Strategic planning
Point-of-care systems, 30
Policy, regulation, and standards, 36, 50, 64
    in CIS organizing framework, 4, 5, 29, 44, 45, 58
    current status, 31–33
    definition of, 4
    historical background, 11–14
    See also Clinical information systems
Practice issues. *See* Professional nursing practice *entries*
Privacy. *See* Data security

Problem-oriented medical record, 20
  See also Data sets; Patient records
Productivity
  computer-based patient record and, 20
  contributors to, 31, 34, 35
  Next Generation criteria, 18, 62
  priority of, 9, 10, 14, 44, 68
Professional nursing practice, 10, 44, 49, 56, 61
  in CIS organizing framework, 4, 5, 58
  current status, 29–31
  historical background, 23–24
  See also Clinical information systems
Professional nursing practice process understanding, 49, 51, 57, 63
  in CIS organizing framework, 4, 5, 29, 44, 58
  definition of, 3
  historical background, 7–11
  See also Clinical information systems
Prototyping, 9, 37, 55
Public key infrastructure (PKI), 33
  See also Data encryption

Q

Quality forums, 14, 31, 32
Quality of care, 54
  contributors to, 31, 32, 35, 44, 47, 50, 53
  Next Generation criteria, 18, 61, 62
  priority of, 16, 30, 33, 68
  See also Patient care

R

Real-time systems, 15, 33, 65
Recruitment, 70, 71
Regulation. *See* Policy, regulation, and standards
Reimbursement, 13, 17, 30
Remote computing. *See* Wireless devices
Research in clinical systems, 45–46, 55, 57
Research Priority Expert Panel on Nursing Informatics (of NCNR), 8–9
Resource management, 9, 10, 32, 34, 37

S

Satellite technology, 33
Scope of Practice for Nursing Informatics, 8, 12–13, 32–33
Shortcuts, 23, 63
  See also Usability
Smart card, 16, 34, 68, 70
Society for Computer Applications in Medical Care (SCAMC), 73–74
Software development, 34, 45, 47, 56
  See also Iterative design; Object-oriented design; Prototyping
Speech recognition. *See* Voice recognition
Standards, 25, 47, 50

data formats, 9, 15, 36, 57, 65
documentation, 24
usability, 21
See also Policy, regulation, and standards
Standards of Practice for Nursing Informatics, 8, 12–13
Steering Committee on Data Bases to Support Nursing Practice. *See under* American Nurses Association
Strategic planning, 11, 13, 36, 69, 70
System design, 4, 24, 29, 58
  iterative, 36, 37
  personnel involved, 38, 45, 47
  process, 51, 52, 56, 57
  redesign, 9, 44, 46, 57
System integration, 14, 32, 33, 43
  across vendors, 36
  Next Generation criteria, 21, 61
  priority of, 16, 17, 68, 69
System utilization, 51
  in CIS organizing framework, 4, 5, 29, 44, 58
  definition of, 4
  historical background, 22–23
  See also Clinical information systems
Systematized Nomenclature of Medicine (SNOMED), 33

T

Taxonomy. *See* Nursing language
Teams and innovation, 9, 46, 47, 56
Technology, 51
  in CIS organizing framework, 4, 5, 29, 44, 58
  definition of, 3–4, 22
  historical background, 14–16
  See also Clinical information systems
Technology adoption
  in CIS organizing framework, 4, 5, 29, 44, 58
  current status, 37–39
  definition of, 4
  historical background, 22–23, 38
  influences outside of health care, 37–39
  See also Clinical information systems
Telemedicine, 16
Terminology. *See* Nursing languages
To Err is Human (IOM 2000), 32
Tool kit technology, 15
Touch screens, 21, 37, 63

U

Unified Medical Language System (UMLS), 8, 73
Unified Modeling Language (UML), 34
  See also Modeling
Unlicensed assistive personnel (UAP), 9
Usability, 36
  concepts, 37
  principles, 22, 63
  See also Error messages; Help features; Human factors; Messaging and alerts; Shortcuts

User interface, 25, 36, 45, 68
    graphical, 15
    requirements, 17, 20, 21, 22–23, 37, 63
    See also Human-computer interaction; Human factors

V

Veterans Health Administration, 35
Vocabulary. *See* Nursing languages
Voice recognition, 15, 35
    data capture via, 21, 37, 63
    priority of, 23, 68, 69, 70

W

Wireless devices, 33, 34, 37, 69, 71
Workflow, 44, 51
    clinical information system support of, 2, 30, 34, 39, 46, 50, 58
Workflow-driven systems, 2, 29, 34, 58
    priority of, 33, 45, 46, 52, 55
    See also under Healthcare information systems: models
World Health Organization (WHO), 23–24
World Wide Web, 16, 31, 33, 37, 70